D1466376

Schizophrenia

———◆———

From Mind to Molecule

AMERICAN PSYCHOPATHOLOGICAL ASSOCIATION SERIES

Schizophrenia

From Mind to Molecule

Edited by

Nancy C. Andreasen, M.D., Ph.D.

Andrew H. Woods Professor
Department of Psychiatry
College of Medicine
Director
Mental Health Clinical Research Center
The University of Iowa Hospitals and Clinics
Iowa City, Iowa

AMERICAN PSYCHOPATHOLOGICAL ASSOCIATION SERIES

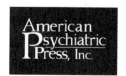

Washington, DC
London, England

Note: The authors have worked to ensure that all information in this book concerning drug dosages, schedules, and routes of administration is accurate as of the time of publication and consistent with standards set by the U.S. Food and Drug Administration and the general medical community. As medical research and practice advance, however, therapeutic standards may change. For this reason and because human and mechanical errors sometimes occur, we recommend that readers follow the advice of a physician who is directly involved in their care or the care of a member of their family.

Copyright © 1994 American Psychiatric Press, Inc.
ALL RIGHTS RESERVED
Manufactured in the United States of America on acid-free paper
First Edition
97 96 95 94   4 3 2 1

American Psychiatric Press, Inc.
1400 K Street, N.W., Washington, DC   20005

Library of Congress Cataloging-in-Publication Data
Schizophrenia : from mind to molecule / edited by Nancy C. Andreasen.
   — 1st ed.
      p.   cm. — (American Psychopathological Association series)
   Includes bibliographical references and index.
   ISBN 0-88048-950-2 (alk. paper)
   1. Schizophrenia. I. Andreasen, Nancy C. II. Series.
   [DNLM: 1. Schizophrenia.   WM 203 S33783 1994]
RC514.S3355   1994   WM
616.89′82–dc20   203
DNLM/DLC   S33783   93-9585
for Library of Congress   1994   CIP

British Library Cataloguing in Publication Data
A CIP record is available from the British Library.

Contents

Contributors ix
Introduction xiii
　Lewis L. Judd, M.D.

Section I
Schizophrenia: The Human Experience

Prologue to Section I 3

1 Schizophrenia: A Parent's Perspective—Mourning
Without End 5
　Martin S. Willick, M.D.

2 Schizophrenia From a Family Point of View:
A Social and Economic Perspective 21
　Laurie M. Flynn

3 Is Biological Psychiatry Building on an Adequate
Base? Clinical Realities and Underlying Processes in
Schizophrenic Disorders 31
　John S. Strauss, M.D.

Section II
The Phenomenology of Schizophrenia

Prologue to Section II 47

4 The Neural Mechanisms of Mental Phenomena 49
　Nancy C. Andreasen, M.D., Ph.D., Victor W. Swayze III, M.D.,
　Michael Flaum, M.D., Daniel S. O'Leary, Ph.D.,
　Randall Alliger, Ph.D.

5 Brain Function in Schizophrenia:
Application of Neurobehavioral Studies 93
   Ruben C. Gur, Ph.D., Andrew J. Saykin, Psy.D.,
   Raquel E. Gur, M.D., Ph.D.

6 Phenomenology, Environmental Risk, and Genetics:
Twin Studies of Schizophrenia 105
   Adrianne M. Reveley, M.D.

Section III
The Neurobiology of Schizophrenia: Traditional Methods and Emerging Technologies

Prologue to Section III 121

7 Postmortem Neurochemical and Neuropathological
Studies in Schizophrenia 123
   James A. Clardy, M.D., Thomas M. Hyde, M.D., Ph.D.,
   Joel E. Kleinman, M.D., Ph.D.

8 Positron-Emission Tomography as a Metabolic and
Neurochemical Probe 147
   Göran Sedvall, M.D., Ph.D.

Section IV
Treatment of Schizophrenia

Prologue to Section IV 159

9 The Search for the Ideal Medications:
Developing a Rational Neuropharmacology 161
   Arvid Carlsson, M.D., Ph.D.

10 Efficacy, Mechanisms, and Side Effects of
Typical and Atypical Neuroleptics 173
   John M. Kane, M.D.

11 Psychosocial Treatments of Schizophrenia:
The Potential of Relationships 189
Thomas H. McGlashan, M.D.

Section V
A Glimpse of the Future:
The Molecular Basis of Schizophrenia

Prologue to Section V 219

12 Molecular Insights Into Schizophrenia 221
Jay W. Pettegrew, M.D., Nancy J. Minshew, M.D.

13 Molecular Genetic Research in Schizophrenia 245
Raymond R. Crowe, M.D.

Index 261

Contributors

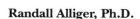

Randall Alliger, Ph.D.
Associate Research Scientist, Mental Health Clinical Research Center, The University of Iowa Hospitals and Clinics, Iowa City, Iowa

Nancy C. Andreasen, M.D., Ph.D.
Andrew H. Woods Professor, Department of Psychiatry, College of Medicine, and Director, Mental Health Clinical Research Center, The University of Iowa Hospitals and Clinics, Iowa City, Iowa

Arvid Carlsson, M.D., Ph.D.
Professor Emeritus, Department of Pharmacology, University of Gothenburg, Gothenburg, Sweden

James A. Clardy, M.D.
Neuropathology Section, Clinical Brain Disorders Branch, Intramural Research Program, National Institute of Mental Health Neuroscience Center at Saint Elizabeths, Washington, D.C.

Raymond R. Crowe, M.D.
Professor, Department of Psychiatry, College of Medicine, The University of Iowa, Iowa City, Iowa

Michael Flaum, M.D.
Assistant Professor, Department of Psychiatry, College of Medicine, The University of Iowa, Iowa City, Iowa

Laurie M. Flynn
Executive Director, National Alliance for the Mentally Ill, Arlington, Virginia

Raquel E. Gur, M.D., Ph.D.
Director, Neuropsychiatry Section, Department of Psychiatry, University of Pennsylvania, Philadelphia, Pennsylvania

Ruben C. Gur, Ph.D.
Director, Brain Behavior Laboratory, Neuropsychiatry Section, Department of Psychiatry, University of Pennsylvania, Philadelphia, Pennsylvania

Thomas M. Hyde, M.D., Ph.D.
Neuropathology Section, Clinical Brain Disorders Branch, Intramural Research Program, National Institute of Mental Health Neuroscience Center at Saint Elizabeths, Washington, D.C.

Lewis L. Judd, M.D.
Director, National Institute of Mental Health, Rockville, Maryland

John M. Kane, M.D.
Chairman, Department of Psychiatry, Hillside Hospital, Division of Long Island Jewish Medical Center, Glen Oaks, New York; and Professor of Psychiatry, Albert Einstein College of Medicine, Bronx, New York

Joel E. Kleinman, M.D., Ph.D.
Neuropathology Section, Clinical Brain Disorders Branch, Intramural Research Program, National Institute of Mental Health Neuroscience Center at Saint Elizabeths, Washington, D.C.

Thomas H. McGlashan, M.D.
Professor of Psychiatry, Yale University School of Medicine; and Chief Executive Officer, Yale Psychiatric Institute, New Haven, Connecticut

Nancy J. Minshew, M.D.
Assistant Professor of Psychiatry and Neurology and Director, Autism and Social Disabilities Program, Department of Psychiatry, Western Psychiatric Institute and Clinic, Pittsburgh, Pennsylvania

Daniel S. O'Leary, Ph.D.
Director, Cognitive Neuroscience Research Unit, Mental Health Clinical Research Center, The University of Iowa Hospitals and Clinics, Iowa City, Iowa

Jay W. Pettegrew, M.D.
Professor of Psychiatry and Neurology and Director,
Neurophysics Laboratory, Department of Psychiatry,
Western Psychiatric Institute and Clinic, Pittsburgh, Pennsylvania

Adrianne M. Reveley, M.D.
Consultant psychiatrist, Maudsley Hospital, London, England

Andrew J. Saykin, Psy.D.
Neuropsychiatry Section, Department of Psychiatry,
University of Pennsylvania, Philadelphia, Pennsylvania

Göran Sedvall, M.D., Ph.D.
Professor and Chairman, Department of Psychiatry and
Psychology, Karolinska Hospital, Stockholm, Sweden

John S. Strauss, M.D.
Professor of Psychiatry, Yale University School of Medicine, New
Haven, Connecticut

Victor W. Swayze III, M.D.
Assistant Professor, Department of Psychiatry, College of Medicine,
The University of Iowa, Iowa City, Iowa

Martin S. Willick, M.D.
Lecturer in Psychiatry, Columbia University College of Physicians
and Surgeons; and Training and Supervising Analyst, New York
Psychoanalytic Institute, New York, New York

Introduction

◆

This volume reflects an exciting moment in the history of schizophrenia research. This costly, devastating, and puzzling disorder is beginning to yield up its long-held secrets to systematic scientific inquiry. We now have the capability to explore, understand, and eventually control the biological foundations of schizophrenia in its myriad forms. It is now unequivocally established that schizophrenia is a brain disorder—possibly one arising very early in development—and we are developing rapidly the scientific and technological sophistication to pinpoint its etiology and the pathophysiological mechanisms that contribute to what most often is a lifelong course.

The pessimism that once permeated both the scientific study of schizophrenia and its clinical treatment has been replaced by a new spirit of excitement and hope that schizophrenia can be understood and conquered within a reasonable time frame. As the chapters of this volume eloquently attest, extraordinary progress is being made in this research field, and even greater accomplishments are expected in the years to come. Even now, before we have fully plumbed the biological substrate of this disorder, today's clinician has available an array of treatments—now augmented significantly by clozapine—that can appreciably improve and normalize the lives of many patients with schizophrenia.

Despite the growing capability of the field, however, substantial knowledge gaps still challenge researchers and clinicians alike, making schizophrenia one of the most pressing public health and research priorities facing the mental health field. Accordingly, the National Institute of Mental Health (NIMH) has launched a broad-based and aggressive schizophrenia research program designed to realize the scientific and clinical potential now visible on the horizon.

In 1988, NIMH completed development of the National Plan for Schizophrenia Research, based on the contributions of 80 leading scientists in the United States and abroad, with an additional 70 scientists serving as advisers and consultants. The plan outlines an intense national research effort to identify the causes of schizophrenia, to develop effective treatments, and to design rational service systems to care for patients with the disease. For more than 2 years we have been implementing the plan while integrating it with the Institute's "Decade of the Brain" plan, a complementary research plan focused on stimulating advances in basic and clinical neuroscience. Activities stemming from the combined plan, known as the National Plan for Research on Schizophrenia and the Brain, are described in the following paragraphs.

NIMH is establishing a variety of research centers that focus on the neuroscience of schizophrenia and other serious mental disorders. To date we have established five Centers for Neuroscience and Schizophrenia, designed to integrate basic and clinical approaches by taking basic research findings from the research laboratory into clinical research settings to improve the diagnosis and treatment of schizophrenia.

More basic neuroscience centers will focus explicitly on molecular neurobiology and will stimulate the application of important genetic and molecular experimental strategies to understand normal and abnormal brain function. In addition, we are launching a major initiative on the molecular genetics of mental illness. NIMH is developing a national "bank" of cell lines from individuals and families with high prevalence of schizophrenia, manic-depressive illness, or Alzheimer's disease. It has also created a network of centers using rigorous, standardized research protocols to identify and meticulously work up informative families and, ultimately, to identify the gene(s) involved. The molecular genetics initiative will include a National Pedigree Research service, which will systematically gather data on large families with many mentally ill members. In addition, a close collaboration has been established with the European Science Foundation's Molecular Genetics Programme. Collectively, these programs will provide the foundation for a coordinated international effort to understand the genetic aspects of schizophrenia and other mental disorders.

To exploit the strong potential of brain imaging to improve our understanding of brain structure and function in schizophrenia and other severe mental disorders, NIMH will soon support up to two positron-emission tomography (PET) centers per year in institutions strong in the clinical sciences, the neurosciences, the cognitive sciences, and neuropsychopharmacology as applied to the study of mental illness.

To improve the knowledge base underpinning the diagnosis, care, and treatment of people with severe and persistent mental disorders such as schizophrenia, NIMH is also mounting a major program to analyze and frame a research agenda for clinical services and services research for such patients. Recognizing the need to link clinical research with service systems research, we have also established the Public-Academic Liaison (PAL) program, designed to foster real partnerships between academic researchers and administrators working in public mental health systems. The goals of this program are to enrich the questions researchers ask by having them conduct their studies in actual service settings, and to foster knowledge transfer to the public service sector through the presence of academic and other researchers.

The ultimate measure of our collective success will be the well-being of the more than 1 million people in the United States with schizophrenia. Theirs is a complex, puzzling, and heterogeneous group of disorders exacerbated by stigma and a service system not structured to respond well to chronic illness. Nonetheless, we expect that initiatives such as those just outlined, coupled with the spontaneous momentum generated by a mental health research field that has at last achieved scientific credibility and distinction equal to any in the biomedical sciences, will yield tangible scientific and clinical progress for these patients and their families in the years to come. A decade hence, if schizophrenia assumes the status of major depression today—a severe but largely manageable disorder—we will regard our efforts as eminently successful.

Lewis L. Judd, M.D.

Section I

Schizophrenia

The Human Experience

Prologue to Section I

Schizophrenia
The Human Experience

———◆———

S chizophrenia is a disease that strikes at the very core of what makes us all human. As the cloud of schizophrenia moves across an individual's horizon, it introduces a barrier between that person and the capacity to experience warmth, to see and think clearly, and to feel and express feelings. The symptoms of schizophrenia run across the entire gamut of capacities that characterize human behavior, cognition, and emotion: perception, thought, language, emotion, volition, and creativity. The capacity to perform these functions well is often replaced by strange and terrifying internal perceptions and experiences, feelings of estrangement, the sense that personal autonomy is being violated, and the sense that control over oneself has been lost. To an outsider, these experiences are often bizarre, frightening, and off-putting. To the person with schizophrenia and his or her family, they are frightening and depressing. The combination of public misconceptions and ignorance with intense internal suffering makes schizophrenia perhaps the most tragic of human illnesses.

The first three chapters in this book express the human experience of schizophrenia from a variety of perspectives. In Chapter 1, Dr. Martin S. Willick presents the human side of schizophrenia as it has been witnessed by the father of a gifted son who developed schizophrenia, a father who also happens to be a gifted psychiatrist. The story of Martin and Gary Willick is reason enough for this book to exist. Dr. Willick eloquently expresses the sense of loss that schizophrenia produces in its victims and their family members. Rarely has this experience been articulated so openly and in such a compelling manner.

In Chapter 2, Laurie M. Flynn, the executive director of the National Alliance for the Mentally Ill (NAMI), presents social and economic perspectives on schizophrenia. Because mental illnesses are poorly understood and therefore often stigmatized, they tend to be poorly funded by state and federal health care agencies. Yet because schizophrenia produces so much long-term disability, patients with this disorder have enormous needs for economic support and social rehabilitative services.

NAMI was organized in the early 1980s to create a public advocacy group that would speak on behalf of seriously mentally ill people. Because many people with schizophrenia are handicapped by their symptoms, they are often unable to speak for themselves. Before NAMI was formed, families tended to be reluctant to discuss the illness of their loved ones. The formation of the NAMI family has provided these family members with an extended support system and a sense of community. In growing strength and numbers, they now actively campaign against stigma and for better health care and improved research funding. The formation of NAMI has been perhaps the most important social force to improve the status of patients with schizophrenia in the past several decades.

In Chapter 3, Dr. John S. Strauss discusses the human side of schizophrenia from the point of view of a research psychiatrist. Dr. Strauss, a well-known and highly admired investigator, provides a thorough critique of clinical research strategies for the study of schizophrenia. Drawing on his many years of experience as both an investigator and a clinician working with people with schizophrenia, he provides wise counsel about the importance of maintaining an open mind, avoiding premature closure, and striking a balance between the study of psychosocial aspects of schizophrenia and its neurobiological aspects.

Chapter 1

Schizophrenia

A Parent's Perspective— Mourning Without End

Martin S. Willick, M.D.

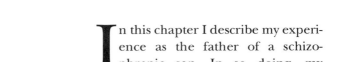

In this chapter I describe my experience as the father of a schizophrenic son. In so doing, my intention is not to tell a tragic story, which of course this is, nor to elicit sympathy, although the families of people devastated by this illness deserve sympathy. Rather, my intention is to present my experience and some reflections on that experience from my perspective as a psychiatrist and psychoanalyst as well as a parent.

Before describing my experience, I wish to emphasize that some of the most intense feelings that I have experienced are also felt by parents of children who have died or who have other kinds of serious illnesses resulting in profoundly impaired functioning. These common feelings are a terrible sense of loss, an ongoing feeling of grief, and a chronic state of mourning, which I have called a mourning without end. But schizophrenia is a unique illness, with extraordinary characteristics that exert their own particular effect on the members of the family. Although many of these characteristics are common to all schizophrenic patients, every case of schizophrenia is in itself unique, so each parent's story will be different. Because of this uniqueness, it is important to provide some background about my son Gary and about the life of our family.

A Personal Story

I have been happily married for 36 years and our family life has been stable with relatively little unhappiness or trauma. There is no mental illness in our immediate families except for a second cousin of mine (incidentally the child of two first cousins who married) who is either schizophrenic or schizoaffective. My wife and I, unfortunately, have had some experience with congenital anomalies, though no one knows whether these are related to schizophrenia. Our first child was a full-term anencephalic girl who died 2 hours after birth. We have had four children since then: Jeffrey, age 30, married, and pursuing a doctorate in astrophysics; Gary, 28, who was born with a congenital anomaly in one eye–the failure of resorption of a small blood vessel in the vitreous of one eye, blocking his central vision—and who has been diagnosed with schizophrenia; Stuart, 27, in medical school; and Karen, 21, a senior in college who was born with a large hemangioma of the chest wall which has since been surgically removed. In our rare moments of speculating about the cause of these congenital anomalies, not to mention schizophrenia, my wife, Nancy, often mentions the fact that she grew up in a small office-apartment in which her father, a dentist, took X rays without any of the precautions currently available.

Two other facts which may or not be relevant concerning etiology are that Gary was born on April 6, placing him among those born in winter or early spring in the Northern Hemisphere; and that when he was 9 months of age he had a viral illness for at least 3 days accompanied by a fever of 106° for much of that time.

Otherwise, his childhood up to his teenage years was, as we say in medicine, "unremarkable." There was, however, something remarkable for us: Gary was a terrific kid, the kind of appealing child that parents feel lucky to have. I say this not to boast but because it is important to understand that the personality of the child who develops schizophrenia will to some extent determine the kind of reactions that parents have. It must be a different experience for parents who have had to struggle with a child who has always had troubles; one who has been shy and schizoid with few friends; or who has had many behavior problems; or who has not been able to get along in school or with peers.

For us, we felt blessed. Gary was personable, empathic, bright, witty, and a wonderful member of the family. He had lots of friends, was quite capable and responsible and very talented. Teachers liked and admired him. Our housekeeper of 20 years says she could always count on him when we were away. But by no means was he a "goody-goody." He was quite capable of being mean to his younger brother, just as his older brother was occasionally mean to him, and he could horse around and exasperate us at times as well.

I often think of these things when I read that a good premorbid personality is one of the factors predictive of a better prognosis. It may be that, in general, the healthier one is before the onset of any illness the better will be the course of that illness. However, for me, the fact that Gary had such a good premorbid personality only means that his illness must be that much more severe to lead to such a devastating outcome. On the other hand, perhaps those admirable premorbid traits that I have described are precisely the ones responsible for the positive aspects of the course of Gary's illness. I will jump ahead of my story a little to say that over the past 10 years Gary has never been violent, has never abused drugs or alcohol, and has been fully compliant with his medication.

If you had been gathering data about him during his senior year of high school, this is what you would have learned: academically, he was ranked first in his class, with a combined score of 1500 on his SATs, and had been accepted to Harvard early decision; he had a close relationship with a girlfriend for 2 years; he was the leader of a jazz group and acknowledged as an outstanding jazz drummer. It is no wonder, then, that he did not go to the 10th reunion of his high school class, because his life has not been the same since his senior year.

I have often been asked, "When did Gary's illness begin?" If I were his psychiatrist writing up the case history, I would say, "when he dropped out of Harvard during his sophomore year" or "at the time of his first hospitalization 2 years later." But when the onset of the illness is so insidious, as it was in Gary's case, and as it is in so many of these young people, it is an impossible question to answer. In retrospect, we have reason to believe that his illness started much earlier.

At age 13, while at summer camp, he became depressed for about a month. At age 14 he asked to see a psychiatrist, whom he saw for 4 years. I later learned that Gary was experiencing certain unusual visual imagery in his fantasy life at that time. Otherwise, the psychiatrist thought he was having some not-untypical adolescent conflicts and never, during the course of those 4 years, had any suspicion of any kind of psychosis. During high school Gary quit the tennis team, saying that he wanted to concentrate on his drumming and band work. At the time it seemed reasonable, but in retrospect it was the beginning of a tendency toward isolation. He asked for a single room at Harvard, although he had always been quite gregarious. During his senior year of high school he sent in his application to Amherst College late; not so unusual for many teenagers, but quite unusual for him.

Here we were, sophisticated parents, knowledgeable about emotional troubles, observant and close to our children, yet we could not see that anything terrible was happening to Gary. He could not decide whether to go to Harvard or Haverford. All kids should have such dilemmas, we thought! After all, I went to Harvard and his older brother was already there. Wasn't it understandable that he would be ambivalent about it? He wanted to be his own person. His well-written college essay was preoccupied with issues of moral integrity and concerns about being phony. Weren't these also concerns appropriate for an adolescent?

It was only when his illness was full-blown that we realized that his ambivalence about his college choice was the early manifestation of the profound ambivalence so characteristic of this illness. At its height he might spend many minutes opening and closing the refrigerator door, each action accompanied by a delusional fear and the attempt to avoid it. Only when his illness was diagnosed did we see that the preoccupation with morality and phoniness which he displayed in his essay was the early form of the typical delusions with which he is still struggling. Despite the fact that these symptoms were already beginning to plague him, he was selected as the leading drummer for the Harvard jazz band during his freshman year and was able to maintain a B average. The next year, however, he could no longer do the work and his condition deteriorated.

Since that time there have been three relatively short hospitalizations, the first of which was necessary because he was suicidal. He had a course of electroconvulsive therapy because the symptoms at that time seemed to be primarily depressive in content. He has been tried on a number of neuroleptics as well as lithium. His last hospitalization, 3 years ago, was to take clozapine. We believe that he was beginning to show some significant improvement on clozapine when he developed agranulocytosis. He is now on loxapine and for the past 2 years has been living not far from us in a halfway house.

What has it been like for us these past 10 years? I will begin with what has always been most painful for me—those feelings of loss, grief, and mourning that I have already mentioned. I feel the loss of the son that I once had, because in many ways he is quite different. Struggling as he does with many of what we now call the "negative symptoms," he has lost that gleam in his eye, that joyous good humor, that zest for life which he once showed. Today, it is hard for him to feel things strongly, or to enjoy his music, sports, or being with the family.

For a long time, when I looked into his eyes I felt that there was no one there. This is one of those manifestations that are difficult for the observer, let alone the person with the illness, to put into words. Some of the expressions that came into my mind were these: "He has become a shell of a person, there is no one there, he has lost his self, he looks different, his face has changed, he's a lost soul."

There has also been a significant cognitive impairment. Things that he was easily able to grasp when he was 14 years old are now much harder for him. He has lost considerable capacity for abstract thinking. His language is very concrete and has lost the richness and subtlety of expression it once had. He has a hard time following a moderately complicated plot of an article he reads or a movie he sees, and he can describe it only in a superficial and concrete way.

I associate these impairments with a certain kind of organicity, a primary impairment of brain functioning, rather than with the distracting effect of his delusions, or with the effect of the neuroleptics, although I am aware that they, too, are exacting their toll. Some manifestations are similar to those I observed in my father-in-law when he developed Alzheimer's disease. When Gary shaves he almost always overlooks some small areas of his face; when he dresses there is almost always something amiss—a shirt not entirely tucked in; a collar not pulled out from under a sweater. He can no longer count on doing those things that most of us do automatically and without thinking when we are dressing.

So we experience this terrible feeling of loss and grieve for the son we knew. There is also that terrible loss of our expectations. We feel cheated out of watching him mature and flower the way adolescents do as they grow into young adults. These feelings are similar to those of people who are in mourning. When I meet his former classmates who are now working, finishing graduate degrees, or married, I am always aware of the fact that these things are not possible for him, just the same as someone would feel had their son died. Yet this mourning is strange, for it is a mourning without an end because, of course, Gary is not dead at all. He is very much still with us, seeming eternally 12 years old, needing constant care and attention.

There is also a loss of a certain kind of emotional connectedness that is a consequence of some of the negative symptoms. These symptoms and the cognitive impairment disturb me much more than they do my wife, who gets more distressed over his delusional thinking. For me, the delusional thinking, as upsetting as it is, is still a sign of lively mental activity,

despite the fact that Gary's thinking is considerably impoverished. I am
more hopeful that the delusions can be altered by medication; I worry
that the cognitive impairment cannot be reversed and that it is associated
with a poorer prognosis. I should add here that there is no doubt whatso-
ever in my mind that neuroleptics do improve the negative symptoms. On
two occasions, Gary was taken off medication. The first time was for the
2-week washout before he took clozapine; the second time was for the 4-
or 5-week period after he developed agranulocytosis. On both occasions,
exactly 9 days after medication was discontinued, he became almost
mute, stopped eating, and was almost totally withdrawn. Although I am
aware that medications also contribute to the negative symptoms, the experience of seeing him off all medication is not one that I ever care to see
again; certainly not until the day comes when he will no longer need it—if
that day ever comes.

This mourning is also strange in that as painful as it is, it coexists with
a lingering hope that one day Gary will be returned to his former self, a
hope strengthened by the improvement on clozapine and the knowledge
that new atypical antipsychotics are not far behind. It is also kindled by
the awareness that two computed tomography (CT) scans, taken several
years apart, have been normal, perhaps indicating that despite the negative symptoms and cognitive impairment, there is no structural change.

A feeling that was present in the early years of his illness was a profound disbelief that this was really happening to him and to us. As young
parents with four children we occasionally worried, like all parents do,
about catastrophes that might befall the children: accidents, leukemia,
brain tumor. We never thought of schizophrenia. For a long time this
sense of disbelief continued, associated with bewilderment. We did not
know what hit us; this could not be happening to him and to us.

Feelings of shame and humiliation can also be a problem for schizophrenic patients and their families. In part this is due to the stigma associated with mental illness, which the National Alliance for the Mentally
Ill is doing everything possible to counteract. Yet there is also some inner
sense of shame or humiliation that I occasionally feel. Why should this be
so? I know that neither I nor Gary has anything to be ashamed of.

An example of a situation that evoked these feelings is a time that I
visited him in the hospital and had to loudly announce my name and
Gary's name and ward to a clerk sitting behind a glass window. Many
other visitors and hospital employees were standing around. I did not
want anyone to hear our name; I had a feeling of shame. I know I would
not have felt the same if he had been on neurology with a brain tumor,

encephalitis, or multiple sclerosis. I also know that it will turn out that his illness is as "organic" as these. Such is the peculiar devastation of mental illness that it evokes such feeling even in someone who should know better. The feeling of humiliation, coupled with the sense of loss, always came to me when I visited him in the hospital. I would think: Gary should be the psychiatric resident here—not the patient!

Although there have been many painful feelings that I have experienced throughout the course of Gary's illness, there have also been some good things. I am proud of my family for the way they have handled all of this. We have stuck together, have been loving and caring, and have kept our own lives happy and productive despite the toll this illness has taken on us. I am proud of my other children, who have stayed loving and supportive despite their own fears and grief. My oldest son, Jeff, now living on the opposite coast, maintains contact with Gary by phone. My son Stuart has been Gary's loyal friend and helper. My daughter, Karen, 7 years younger than Gary, has courageously made every effort to maintain the close and loving relationship she had with him before he became ill. Both of them are much better than my wife and I in helping Gary to feel normal and one of the kids. Perhaps our disappointment and anguish is more obvious to him than is theirs. Although each of my children has his or her own anguished story about the experience of having a brother with schizophrenia, I am proud that despite all that we have been through, we have been able to support each other.

I have also been fortunate in having close friends who have been loyal and understanding. We have been fortunate, too, in having good psychiatrists and mental health professionals taking care of Gary. I have encountered only one physician who did not treat us well, and our contact with him was rather short-lived. I have no horror stories to tell about bad treatment and inconsiderate doctors, nurses, or aides, although I have heard these complaints from others. No one has blamed us for his illness as was the case for parents of schizophrenic children some years ago.

I know that I should be most proud of Gary, and I can often feel that. The problem is that it is not easy to see that he is displaying great courage in coping with what has happened to him. The symptoms of the illness make him appear lacking in motivation, initiative, and will, and even he accuses himself of not trying hard enough. It is hard for an observer to see how difficult it must be for him to get up every day, hoping to feel different, only to awake with the same feeling of anhedonia. In some ways, those admirable qualities that he possessed before he became ill are no doubt still serving him well as he tries to fight an illness that none of us, let alone Gary himself, can really comprehend.

We have also come to a point of greater stability in his illness. For many years we lived in fear of the next hospitalization, the further deterioration, and, most importantly, the fear of his suicide. Alongside of our feelings of anguish were many days, weeks, and months of constant anxiety. For a number of years, and even now to a certain extent, we were not free to come and go, to take vacations, or to go out on the spur of the moment. He has been living in a halfway house since 1988. He drives his car every day to a center for work rehabilitation. He has been playing his drums again, and has begun to work with some programs on his computer. We are hoping that the next step is an apartment; after that, a part-time job. It is, of course, not what we expected years ago, but we are grateful for the improvement. All the members of the family have come to a painful but better feeling of acceptance of Gary. This acceptance has gradually replaced the acute sense of anguish, disappointment, anger, and despair that we felt for a number of years. This change is good for all of us, including Gary. It is clear to me that in patients who develop the chronic form of the illness, the acute phase can last not just a few months or a year but as many as 5–10 years.

A Clinician's Perspective

In the remainder of this chapter I discuss some concepts related to schizophrenia from the perspective of a psychiatrist and psychoanalyst who is also the parent of a schizophrenic patient. This discussion is based on my readings as well as on my many discussions with patients, families, and colleagues.

Nonresponders

I want to briefly discuss the concept of nonresponders. Gary has been called by some psychiatrists a nonresponder to neuroleptics. Three different classes of these drugs have not done away with his delusions, hallucinations, or negative symptoms. However, he is at least a partial responder, as was so painfully evident when he was taken off all medication. We can legitimately say someone is a nonresponder only if there is no difference between the medicated and the nonmedicated state. In addition, in Gary's case, reducing his medication, which has proved to be effective in so many schizophrenic patients, is very detrimental. He has consistently been extremely sensitive to even small reductions, with an obvious exacerbation of symptoms.

Overinvolvement and Expressed Emotion

I have been interested in the area of psychosocial education because our family, and especially our children, were helped by this approach. It is very important for the family to understand what is happening to their child and sibling so that they will be better able to provide a supportive and caring environment. In this connection the work of Leff and Vaughn (1985) on overinvolvement and expressed emotion clearly has been important. However, I have a mixed reaction to the use of these concepts.

There is no doubt in my mind that helping the family to understand schizophrenia can prevent exacerbations of the illness. But there is something about these terms that is absurd. What is absurd is this: How can a loving parent of a schizophrenic child be anything else but "overinvolved"? The illness and the incapacity it brings with it require the parents to once more be involved with the care and guidance of a child who most likely had already demonstrated his independence and initiative. Gary was our most independent and efficient child; schizophrenia robbed him of his independence and self-hood.

It is true that once the illness has begun to abate, parents must give their child the encouragement and freedom to resume the growth and development that was so cruelly arrested. At this juncture, parents may need help in relinquishing their involvement to some degree consistent with the progress of their child. I hope that this is what is really meant by the attempt to reduce overinvolvement.

The concept of "expressed emotion," which primarily refers to being excessively critical, also has some merit. However, once again there is something absurd about the idea as much as it is true. During the early phases of the illness, no normal family can contain their critical feelings because the symptomatic manifestations are so similar to many behaviors that any parent would be critical of. It must be understood that critical feelings during this stage are unavoidable and do not give any indication of how loving and devoted a family has been. Once it has become clear that one is dealing with schizophrenia, it is essential that the family understand that much of the behavior that distresses them is beyond the patient's control and is due to an illness. But even when this is understood, it is not always easy to tame one's critical feelings in the face of paranoid rages or the absence of demonstrable affection, which are characteristic symptoms of this illness. This is, of course, also true for families who deal with relatives with Alzheimer's disease or brain damage due to trauma.

Etiology

It is hard to sit with a family affected by schizophrenia without getting into some discussion about etiology. I have recently been trying to educate some psychoanalysts who still cling to notions about the schizophrenogenic mother or the effect of early parental neglect in this illness. It is not that I doubt that there are infants at risk for profound mental disturbance due to impaired upbringing. There are many serious psychiatric disorders that are primarily caused by parental abuse and neglect without a primary biological abnormality. Therefore, I do not agree with many members of the National Alliance for the Mentally Ill who divide the mentally ill into only two categories: those with biological mental illnesses and the "worried well."

To the best of our knowledge, schizophrenia is a biological illness, but there is still a great deal of controversy about the complexity of the etiology. The illness certainly does not follow a simple hereditary model such as is found in Huntington's chorea. Just as we were becoming more convinced by the adopted-away studies that environment plays a minor role in the etiology of the illness, a Finnish study (Tienari et al. 1987) concluded that healthy family rearing is a protective factor in the children given up for adoption by schizophrenic mothers. So we fall back on the idea that the illness is heterogeneous with multiple etiologies, including biological, psychological, and social factors.

I do not doubt that psychological and social factors play a role in many serious mental illnesses and certainly in personality development in general. These factors can also have a profound influence on the course of the illness and its personal, particular manifestations. However, I seriously doubt that anything but a biological disturbance, whether genetic or viral, is the basic cause of Gary's illness. When I reflect on these matters I sometimes try to imagine, comparing the situation to that which currently exists for Huntington's disease, what would have happened had we had a test that showed us that Gary had the potential to be schizophrenic. What sort of upbringing could we have devised that would have placed minimal stress on him to prevent the illness from occurring?

Other than bringing him up in an entirely different kind of society, it is hard to imagine what kind of preventive measures to reduce stress would have been useful. As a matter of fact, most of those that I can think of probably would have been detrimental to the growth and development that he did achieve. For example, we might not have allowed him to go to sleep-away camp when he was 8 years old because we would have been fearful of the consequences of the separation. Yet this was a wonderful experience for him, and he did not have any problems with it. Perhaps we would have thought of sending him to private school, with smaller classes and more attention. But he thrived in public school, had many friends who liked and admired him, and did well without great difficulties. Should he not have started to date a girl at age 15, joined the tennis team, become the leader of a teenage jazz band, studied hard to maintain his A average? All of these things enriched his life and solidified his sense of himself prior to the onset of the serious manifestations of his illness.

I raise these questions because the effects of psychological, social, and environmental stresses are often discussed in relation to the etiology of schizophrenia. But these stresses are a part of any child's life. If, armed with the knowledge of a possible future schizophrenic illness, we had planned to intervene, it probably would not have altered anything and might very well have done some harm. In retrospect, it seems to me that he should not have gone to Harvard. But the truth is, his illness had already begun and we did not realize it.

There is no doubt that once the illness has manifested itself, stressful situations must be reduced. These can, no doubt, have an effect on the course of the illness, just as the family's behavior has an effect. For many cases, however, these factors may play a minor role in the etiology of the disease. Perhaps for many other cases, which may have a different etiology, they do make an important contribution.

Delusions

Psychoanalysts pay a great deal of attention to the content of delusions in an attempt to understand not only the experience of the patient, but perhaps the origins of the illness as well. In most instances that is not as useful as using medication to do away with the delusions, but one approach does not contradict the other. I believe that many of the thought disturbances we call delusions are the schizophrenic patient's attempt to explain or to put into words what his or her experience is.

For example, Gary now is plagued by the delusion that he has lost his heart. He frequently asks people if they think this is possible. At times he will acknowledge that he knows he cannot live without having his heart, the organ that pumps blood throughout the body, and he says it must be his spiritual heart that he has lost. At other times he returns to the concrete idea that it is his physical heart, for he no longer feels it beating or pounding upon exertion.

For many years before the onset of this delusion, Gary used other language to describe what he was experiencing. He said he couldn't get into anything, he couldn't get into his music, he was bad because he couldn't feel his previous affection for us. These expressions coincided with the increased flattening of affect, the loss of feeling that is such a pathognomonic feature of this illness. So, what Gary is saying is essentially correct—he has lost some of that capacity to feel strong emotions which all of us attribute, in our metaphoric way, to our heart, even though it is a function of our brain. But for Gary it is not a metaphor; it is as real to him as anything else. We call it a delusion or false belief, although, in another sense, what he is saying is true—he has lost his heart. We accept it as a metaphor for his emotional experience; he experiences it in a concrete way with a literal meaning.

Advice for Clinicians

As a result of my personal and professional experiences, I can offer some advice to practicing clinicians. This advice may be familiar but it is worth repeating. First, clinicians should listen to families of schizophrenic patients as they tell their story and their observations. Use them to guide you in your recommendations, including the use of medications. The members of our family are always the first to notice alterations in Gary's condition. We see them much before Gary does and often before the treating psychiatrist does. When medication has been changed or the dose altered, we are the most reliable observers of the changes that are taking place. I mentioned earlier that I had only one unfortunate experience with a psychiatrist, who was the head of an inpatient unit. He did not care to listen to our opinion and, as a matter of principle, did not encourage his residents to speak with the families; he left that task to the social worker.

In most instances, young schizophrenic patients are still living at home with their families. The families, therefore, must be included in the treatment program. In those instances where the patient resides in a halfway house or supervised apartment, the mental health professionals involved in the patient's care should be given training in understanding the symptoms and manifestations of the illness and ways to help the patients cope with them.

Another important issue is rehabilitation. There is a critical need for housing and alternative living arrangements for schizophrenic patients. Ideally, every inpatient unit should have an aftercare program that includes a gradual transition to the community. As far as other aspects of rehabilitation are concerned, my experience has led me to consider two possibilities. One possibility is the increased input of neuropsychologists, who might begin to help patients deal with their cognitive impairment to see if relearning can take place with some forms of assistance. It has been shown that patients who do not do well initially on the Wisconsin Card Sorting Test (Heaton 1985) can do better with some rewards and instruction (Green et al. 1990). Perhaps the experience of psychologists who have worked in this area with head trauma victims could be of benefit to us as well.

A second possibility is the use of the computer for training and relearning. Software programs could be devised to enhance social skills as well as to teach patients a particular occupation, such as bookkeeping. For those patients who are able to concentrate to a sufficient degree, the computer offers a number of benefits. It can be used when one is alone, without the distractions of a surrounding crowd of people. It can be done at one's own pace, with time to go over things not easily comprehended.

The most important task that lies ahead is to develop the tools to understand the etiology and pathogenesis of schizophrenia and to develop new medications that will be even more beneficial than those that we have now. We are on the right track with clozapine, but we must find similar drugs that do not carry the risk of agranulocytosis.

When I heard about the risk of agranulocytosis, I never gave it a second thought because the risk was so small and the possibility for significant improvement far outweighed this risk. Many patients and families are experiencing a kind of living death anyway; therefore it was a risk worth taking. But the experience of getting agranulocytosis, even though it is not fatal, can be a formidable one. In Gary's case, not only was he taken off all medication for 4 or 5 weeks, but he was placed in isolation on a medical service. The isolation itself was probably not very helpful, and it took him a long time to recover psychologically. I think a clinician should spend some time not only spelling out the risk of getting agranulocytosis, but also explaining to the patient and the family what is likely to happen if the patient does develop this unfortunate side effect.

Concluding Comments

Perhaps it is fitting for me as a psychoanalyst to end this chapter by describing a dream that I had and the events of the preceding day that stimulated some of its content—what we call the day residue. I was, along with a colleague of mine, giving an all-day Saturday colloquium at Mount Sinai Hospital in New York on psychoanalytic perspectives on borderline personality disorder. The night before, the coordinator of the colloquium called to say that he would have to miss the morning session but would meet us for lunch. At the luncheon he somewhat sheepishly explained that he had chosen to attend his young son's basketball game instead of our presentation. My colleague said that he could readily understand that, and then, referring to me, said, "Marty can certainly appreciate that, since he has never gotten over his oldest son's hitting a home run with two out in the ninth to win a championship baseball game." That night I had the following dream.

> I was sitting in the stands at a championship baseball game much as I had done on that day, 15 years ago, when my son Jeff, who was the baseball player, had hit the home run. But in the dream the batter at the plate was Gary, not Jeff. It was also two out in the ninth, a runner on base, and the team was behind by one run. Gary then hit a long line drive home run, similar to the one I had seen that day, but also similar to those I had often seen during my boyhood at Ebbets Field where the Brooklyn Dodgers used to play. As Gary rounded third base and everyone was cheering, I saw that he was "cured" of his schizophrenia. He had that wonderful expression on his face that I loved and remembered. I saw that everyone else was cheering because they, too, knew that he was cured. During the real game 15 years ago, as Jeff rounded third base in front of where I had been sitting, I had run down the stands shouting, as I relived my boyhood hero fantasies, "He did it, he did it." In the dream, I ran down the stands shouting at the top of my lungs about Gary, "He's cured, he's cured.'"

Then . . . I woke up!

My hope is that clinicians and researchers will continue their efforts to treat schizophrenia more effectively and, ultimately, to find a cure for it, so that my dream, and the dream of so many others, will come true.

References

Green MF, Ganzell S, Satz P, et al: Teaching the Wisconsin Card Sorting Test to schizophrenic patients (letter). Arch Gen Psychiatry 47:91–92, 1990

Heaton R: Wisconsin Card Sorting Test. Odessa, TX, Psychological Assessment Resources, 1985

Leff J, Vaughn C: Expressed Emotion in Families. New York, Guilford, 1985

Tienari P, Sorri A, Lahti I, et al: Genetic and psychosocial factors in schizophrenia. Schizophr Bull 13:477–485, 1987

Chapter 2

Schizophrenia From a Family Point of View

A Social and Economic Perspective

Laurie M. Flynn

———◆———

To adequately consider a social and economic perspective on schizophrenia, it is necessary to identify several unique characteristics of this group of severely mentally ill people. The most significant feature is the often extreme degree of disability that accompanies severe mental disorders, especially schizophrenia. Current goals for the care and treatment of persons with schizophrenia focus on maintenance of functioning and rehabilitation. This focus assumes that schizophrenia represents long-term disability in which important goals such as increasing independence and enhancing social adjustment, as well as meeting basic human needs, are all vital. However, attainment of these goals is complicated by the high incidence of poverty among individuals with schizophrenia. Poverty is the most pervasive characteristic of adults afflicted with schizophrenia.

Another important characteristic of persons with schizophrenia is

I want to thank the organizers of this book, and especially Dr. Nancy Andreasen, for including the family perspective in their overview of schizophrenia. This acknowledgment of the importance of family, both in individual cases and in the larger realm of policy and public life, is much appreciated.

their near-total reliance on public mental health services. The number of persons with mental disabilities such as schizophrenia, and specifically excluding mental retardation, who have enrolled in the federal supplemental security income (SSI) and supplemental security disability income (SSDI) programs rose astronomically during the 1980s. The Social Security Administration in 1989 reported a increase of 44% in the number of SSI recipients who have a primary mental disorder. Similarly, the number of SSDI recipients with a mental disability has increased by an astonishing 67.5% since 1984, as reported by Lave and Goldman. Public hospitals and general hospital psychiatric units in the United States now treat a disproportionate number of indigent patients with schizophrenia. Publicly supported clinics, residential programs, and rehabilitation programs are currently the main source of care for a majority of persons with schizophrenia and other serious mental illnesses. The Medicaid program is now the largest single source of federal support for the care of severely mentally ill individuals, nearly all of them with a diagnosis of schizophrenia. This is a striking shift from earlier policies, which relied almost exclusively on state hospital care.

A major feature of the problems facing individuals with schizophrenia relates to the broad range of social, human, and medical services that now constitute state-of-the-art treatment. Virtually all mentally ill individuals and their families must negotiate a fragmented and frustrating set of programs, providers, and government bureaucracies. Complying with difficult treatment regimens; obtaining and remaining in adequate, affordable housing; applying for and maintaining various entitlements; and participating in other vital programs such as vocational rehabilitation are all obstacles that frequently confront and confound persons with schizophrenia. As one witty physician noted at the 1988 national convention of the National Alliance for the Mentally Ill (NAMI), "We now have a mental health system based on scheduled appointments trying to reach a client population that doesn't own watches." While the intent of community mental health centers was certainly laudable, it seems clear that in many parts of the country they have failed to meet their basic goals. The seriously mentally ill, made up largely of those with a diagnosis of schizophrenia, are poor by policy design. They have long-term and complex needs, which must be adequately met if they are to live in the community. Yet these individuals, because of their disability and ongoing lack of social support, often function very poorly in the role of consumer. Most cannot function well enough to demand, maintain, and monitor the services they require.

Not surprisingly, a related problem, which has become more acute in recent years, is the rising tide of indigence among seriously mentally ill people. Persons with schizophrenia and other severe mental illnesses are overrepresented among the medically indigent and the uninsured. Patients diagnosed with serious mental disorders are a major source of uncompensated hospital care. While the origins of this problem are many, perhaps the most significant is the disruption in an individual's life imposed by the onset of schizophrenia. Persons with schizophrenia are downwardly mobile, and the loss of income and poor prospects for future earnings and gainful employment become part of the distress inherent in the disease. The American Psychiatric Association has well documented the gaps in private insurance for mental disorders that contribute to the indigence of persons with schizophrenia. Members of NAMI see these policies as simple discrimination against a particular class of patients.

Public Policy Issues

One of the most difficult public policy issues facing those concerned about the care of people with schizophrenia is the allocation of resources across the various treatment settings. For the past two decades, a consensus has been emerging that most severely mentally ill people can be successfully treated in the community at a cost that is comparable to that of caring for such patients in mental hospitals. This consensus on the part of families and professionals reflects our experience with the continued expansion of care for seriously mentally ill individuals in community settings, and the ongoing implementation of deinstitutionalization. It is now estimated that fully 80% of individuals with schizophrenia and other long-term mental illnesses spend most of their time in noninstitutional community settings. Although there is general agreement that community settings are appropriate and therapeutic for nearly all individuals with schizophrenia, state mental health budgets continue to allocate a majority of funds to public mental institutions. Approximately 65% of the budgets of state mental health agencies, according to the National Association of State Mental Health Directors, is currently spent to support state mental hospitals. Although nearly everyone agrees that this budget share is too large, it has proved difficult if not politically dangerous to rapidly reallocate these large resources. Local political realities, the continued need for quality hospital care for some patients, union issues, retraining of workers, and the inadequacy of connections between inpatient and outpatient services have all made transformation of the resources a very difficult challenge.

The structure and administration of the Medicaid program and related federal entitlement programs create particular problems in financing the care of individuals with serious mental illness. Approximately 50% of individuals with schizophrenia are enrolled in the federal SSI program. However, there is little incentive for public providers who are deficit funded to assist potentially eligible individuals to enroll. Gaps in access to entitlements and difficulties in blending funding sources also contribute to indigence among mentally ill people. Fragmentation and discrimination create severe problems for individuals who are truly disabled and need ongoing care and treatment.

The rise of homelessness among the mentally ill is perhaps the most highly publicized side effect of massive deinstitutionalization. The Urban Institute estimated several years ago that as many as one-third to one-half of the homeless persons in the United States are individuals with a significant history of psychiatric disorders. A conservative estimate is that as many as 200,000 of the nation's mentally ill citizens are now drifting in urban centers from shelters to streets and, unfortunately, even to jails. The Medicaid program, which is the major source of financial support for individuals with schizophrenia, has been under increasing pressure from both federal and state legislatures to contain its explosive growth. Concerns about rising health care costs have led to the adoption of policies that restrict access for individuals with mental illness and do not recognize the unique characteristics of this population and the treatment techniques that serve them best. The most serious consequence has been a lack of willingness to expand definitions of reimbursable services to accommodate recent community-based innovations in care. Case management and psychosocial rehabilitation, for example, are available only as "optional" services. Consequently, they are not usually covered under state Medicaid programs and frequently are not available to those who need them the most. Where these services are covered, the reimbursement levels are so low that providers find payment levels inadequate and are unwilling to participate in the programs.

State Medicaid programs tend to structure reimbursements in such a way as to encourage institutional care over community-based treatment. The state budget absorbs the cost of treatment in state hospitals; only outpatient care is covered by Medicaid. In part, this is due to concerns over management of cost increases. The result, however, is that prices for hospital care tend to more closely approximate the actual cost of care than fees set for community providers. Eligibility for Medicaid is linked to institutional treatment. This occurs partly because of spend-down provisions, and regulations governing eligibility. Families are all too familiar with these provisions, which force them to use all of their available resources, even to mortgage their homes and deplete their savings, to support their relative in dire need of immediate help. If families provide additional cash, an automobile, rent, or any other support to their mentally ill relative, the value of such support is deducted from the amount of support received through federal entitlement programs. Current levels of support do not allow a life of dignity in most communities, yet families are penalized if they do what comes naturally and provide supplementary income of in-kind support. Clearly, individuals with schizophrenia are very poorly served by our publicly financed mental health and welfare systems.

A New Approach

Against this grim background it is exciting to see the rise of the family/consumer movement, a new impact on the social and economic lives of individuals with schizophrenia. This is an area in which advocacy has long been needed. Over the past two decades, psychiatry has witnessed a profound change in the paradigm underpinning our notions about schizophrenia. To summarize briefly, we have moved from understanding the origins of mental illness as being principally psychodynamic to appreciating the basic biological component of the disease. The locus of care for persons with schizophrenia has changed as well. We formerly relied almost exclusively on long-term care in large mental institutions. Now more than 80% of such individuals are living in the community. Previously professionals viewed their role in providing care for persons with schizophrenia as being one of protection and custody. Today we seek larger goals of normalization and rehabilitation; mainstreaming for this population is now encouraged. For several hundred years, the medical profession had almost an exclusive role in defining care needs and making treatment decisions. Today we see the rising importance of self-help, and we see the increasing impact of cost control in all medical decision making. For many years, we responded to people with schizophrenia best when they were in need of acute care and treatment. Today we increasingly focus resources on maintenance, wellness, and prevention of relapse. Families have gone, in 20 years, from being treated as part of the problem to being actively invited onto the treatment team as part of the solution.

The Costs of Schizophrenia

Although we know much about the syndrome of schizophrenia, only in the past decade have we begun to measure effectively the true cost of this devastating illness. In 1988, mental illness cost Americans $129.7 billion. Of this amount, $57 billion—or 44% of the total—was the cost of lost productivity and $55.4 billion—or 43% of the total—was spent on medical care. The value of time spent caring for mentally ill family members and the cost of crime and associated criminal justice system expenditures related to mental illness amounted to nearly $6 billion.

Studies done by the National Institute of Mental Health (NIMH) indicate that as much as 15% of the population—or 27 million Americans over age 18—will experience a mental disorder within any given 6-month period; of this total, only about 1%–1.5% will have the diagnosis of schizophrenia. Approximately 2.7 million individuals over the course of a lifetime will be diagnosed and treated for schizophrenia. What is most important is that this relatively small number of individuals will account for more than three-fourths of the total amount spent by taxpayers for the care and treatment of mental illnesses, and more than 90% of the lost productivity ratio. For most people with severe schizophrenia, being a patient is their only career.

The reference to the cost of medical care should be understood to include the physical disorders that often go undiagnosed in schizophrenic individuals. Nearly one-half of the patients in one large state mental hospital were found, upon examination, to have significant physical disease, and almost none of them were receiving adequate treatment. One consumer said to me several years ago, "The medical profession appears to feel that if I have been diagnosed with schizophrenia, there is nothing below my neck that they need to be concerned about."

The reference to the cost associated with the criminal justice system reflects a horrifying phenomenon perhaps less well understood than it should be. Much of what we have called "deinstitutionalization" of seriously mentally ill individuals is, in fact, "transinstitutionalization." A rising tide of schizophrenic and other severely disordered individuals are now being seen in American jails. Having an untreated mental illness is being

treated as a criminal activity. These helpless persons are arrested for mis-
demeanor offenses such as disorderly conduct and trespass, and are
languishing in jails in increasing numbers. Jails have, in fact, become the
new asylums as many police departments feel that it is more humane to
arrest severely mentally ill people than to leave them outdoors where they
risk freezing to death under bridges or in city parks. Today, we have more
seriously mentally ill individuals in the Los Angeles County Jail than in all
five California mental hospitals combined. In fact, the Los Angeles
County Jail has more mentally ill individuals than the nation's largest
state hospital. The Miami, Florida, jail houses more than 1,800 mentally
ill inmates each month, living in dreadful conditions while the state
legislature decides not to fund expansion at two overcrowded state facilities.

Societal costs are tremendous, but even more difficult to measure are
the costs of schizophrenia to families. These hidden, personal costs are
no less real. Families experience an incredible devastation in their personal lives as they see a beloved relative become a stranger. Social relationships, marital relationships, and the health of other family members
are all severely strained. We are only beginning to understand the impact
on siblings whose family life is so distorted by the overwhelming needs of
the severely ill brother or sister. Not infrequently, families react with
anger, shame, denial, and isolation. The stigma of mental illness has been
reduced somewhat over the past decade, but is still so strong that many
find it difficult to say "schizophrenia" out loud, even to close relatives and
neighbors.

Another hidden problem of unknown dimensions is the increasing
incidence of violence within the family. Severely ill people with schizophrenia who may not be consistently compliant with treatment regimens
are often difficult to manage at home. Families report that threats and
actual incidents of violence are a constant companion in their daily lives,
and yet they must enter into a distasteful and adversarial involuntary commitment process if they wish any protection or relief. All too often, this
process demeans everyone involved and results in only short-term intervention.

The stress, the heartbreak, and the incredible pain of having a relative living in one's home with this devastating illness create enormous
ongoing disruptions in family life. Even with the advent of family support
groups and the vital coping skills and the education that these groups
offer, families report tremendous loss associated with schizophrenia—
loss of their dreams, loss of control in their personal and financial lives,

loss of independence as they assume the burden of years of caregiving, and often loss of vital personal relationships as other members of the family withdraw. Who can truly assess the costs to a family that sees its dreams and hopes for a cherished young person perish under the weight of severe mental illness?

Families worry, too, about the long-term impact of schizophrenia and the failed governmental health policies. They look at the national disgrace of the homeless and worry that their relative may soon be among this unfortunate army. Indeed, the homeless mentally ill are our nation's "untouchables," hallucinating in doorways, hiding under bridges, crouching in the shadows of our cities. Homeless mentally ill individuals diminish our spirit, wound our personal dignity, and increase our nation's shame as we confront what seems to be an intractable problem. For families, this problem has a name and a face—and is a loved relative. "What will happen after I am gone, and there is no one to pick up the pieces?" is the plaintive cry of many NAMI members. It is important that we apply the full power of America's best resources to bringing order out of the billions of dollars' worth of chaos in annual public funds for care and treatment of schizophrenia. We must recall the fact that suicide is currently the major cause of death for young schizophrenic individuals, and that the number of seriously mentally ill individuals without any support at all continues to grow.

Proposed Actions

There are some solutions that should be implemented to begin to assist in providing appropriate care and treatment for schizophrenic individuals. These solutions have been suggested by policymakers in the family movement.

First, recognize that schizophrenia is a brain disease and accord it equal status with all other diseases. This means setting a priority in state mental health programs on schizophrenia, because these individuals are far and away the most disabled and neediest of the population requiring assistance. It also means an end to discrimination in public and private insurance programs, recognizing that schizophrenia is truly an illness, and may not be covered as a second-class "psychological" problem.

Second, end the fiscal shell game, whereby the state and federal governments continue to deny responsibility for the full range of treatment needed by individuals with schizophrenia. We must recognize that making seriously mentally ill people eligible for federal support such as SSI, SSDI, and Medicaid has effectively divided the fiscal responsibility for their care. We have, in fact, set up conflicting rules and decisions about care, driven almost entirely by financial concerns. We could rectify this situation immediately by taking all federal funds currently allocated to the treatment of mentally ill people and redistributing them in the form of block grants to state mental health authorities. Alternatively, we might create an entirely new federal mental illness entitlement, giving maximum flexibility to the state and requiring the state to take full responsibility not only for medical care, but also for vital rehabilitation, housing, and ongoing social and economic support of these disabled individuals.

Third, recognize that existing psychiatric human resources must be utilized more effectively to treat people with schizophrenia in the community. There is no shortage of trained psychiatrists, psychologists, and social workers in the United States; in fact, the mental health professions have grown remarkably in the past several decades. However, almost without exception we find that these professionals specialize in counseling and psychotherapy, preferring to work with those who are less severely ill than patients with schizophrenia. They clearly also prefer to work with patients covered by third-party reimbursement, which is more generous than state and federal programs. Yet almost all professionals were trained in part using public funds. Such training programs at university and postgraduate levels should require a payback obligation on a one-for-one basis that will require the mental health professional to work in the public sector with severely mentally ill people. This one action alone would dramatically improve the access to care of this most disadvantaged patient group. It has even been suggested that such public service should continue after the payback obligation, as part of an ongoing pro bono requirement of public service for continued state licensure. Whatever course is chosen, we must find a way to bring our best-trained professionals into the challenge of caring for severely mentally ill patients with schizophrenia.

Finally, continue to increase federal support for research on schizophrenia. The publication in 1986 by NIMH of "The National Plan for Schizophrenia Research" was a landmark, but we have far to go to implement its wide-ranging set of recommendations. Schizophrenia is still dramatically underfunded when compared with funds for research on heart and lung disease (over $1 billion each, every year) or cancer (over $1.5 billion per year). The rapid increase in funding for acquired immunodeficiency syndrome (AIDS) should give us all an important lesson in the value of the research community joining with the advocacy community to increase the priority placed on solving the riddle of schizophrenia and other severe mental illnesses.

Until we do find the cause and cure for schizophrenia, the realities and the burdens of the social and economic costs of this most devastating of all mental disorders will remain with us. As family members, we recognize the need for aggressive advocacy across all fronts: policy, program, and research. Both biomedical research and vital research on service innovations and treatment interventions are needed. Only with a partnership approach can we hope to achieve the results we are all seeking on behalf of individuals with schizophrenia—the day when all suffering is ended and schizophrenia is part of medical history.

Chapter 3

Is Biological Psychiatry Building on an Adequate Base?

Clinical Realities and Underlying Processes in Schizophrenic Disorders

John S. Strauss, M.D.

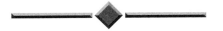

T he 1990s have been called the Decade of the Brain, and the dominant efforts in psychiatry currently are focused on discovering biological causes of mental illness. But this endeavor may be building on an inadequate base, attempting to develop biological explanations for phenomena that in reality are secondary processes or are descriptively quite different from what they are assumed to be. Just as it is not wise in science to carry out mathematical calculations from empirical data to decimal points more precise than measurement error permits, in psychiatry today it is very possible that progress in the neurosciences will be severely limited by major short-

This report is supported in part by NIMH Grants MH00340 and MH34365 and by a grant from the National Association for Research in Schizophrenia and Depression (NARSAD).

comings in descriptive psychiatry and the concepts it uses, the clinical data to which the biological findings must ultimately relate.

The Biological Versus the Psychodynamic Approach

The possibility that progress in the neurosciences will be limited by shortcomings in descriptive psychiatry is suggested by the recent history of psychiatry. Descriptive diagnostic and outcome studies have been eagerly sought by biological psychiatrists who felt a strong need to get beyond the vague classification systems of previous years to more reliable diagnoses (e.g., Strauss and Carpenter 1975). For psychiatrists trained psychodynamically who desired a science more careful about the simple but basic notions of proof and measurement, descriptive psychiatry also offered a longed-for objectivity. The psychodynamic literature had frequently made assumptions about the definitive nature of "what I showed in my last paper." Psychodynamic reports, even those of classical importance, often attended little to classification, using words such as "psychosis" and "schizophrenia" interchangeably.

But in the history of human endeavors steady progression is a rarity. Rather we tend to lurch back and forth from one extreme approach to the opposite. In psychiatry, increased attention to measurement, classification, and biology has been associated with the narrowing of focus to patient characteristics that can be readily measured and to categorizing these in dichotomous ways. This emphasis has involved failure to attend to phenomena that may be important but are difficult to assess reliably.

This neglect in turn is often bolstered by the belief that finally a more balanced approach has been achieved. This belief is a kind of historicism—those who came before did not get it right but we have now—and is reminiscent of the previous era. Psychiatric residencies that used to have a heavy psychodynamic emphasis also often prided themselves on their balanced approaches. Sometimes when a resident raised the possibility of a biological contribution to a particular disorder, a supervisor might say, "Yes, there probably is a constitutional factor," and then move back to psychodynamics, leaving the feeling that one was being eclectic and reasonable. In retrospect, the word "constitutional" seems often to have been considered adequate to cover and dispense with genetics, brain structure, physiologic mechanisms, and any one of a number of other fields that are now viewed as separate domains with their own body of knowledge. In those days, "balance" was also often a few rooms and a couple of biologists doing research, when the rest of the hospital was focused on psychodynamics.

These statements are made not to blame the efforts of the past, but to suggest that the field has a tendency to deal with diversity in a rather characteristic fashion irrespective of the particular content area that is being emphasized or neglected. Now in discussions of severe psychopathology, one often hears "that was stress," in which the word "stress" is treated as an adequate notion covering the field, just as "constitutional" used to be. That quick disposition occurs in spite of the diverse nature and complexities of "stress" (e.g., Rutter 1981). The use of the concept "demoralization" these days often has a similar role. And the word "psychosocial" is a particularly good example of the way in which our language tells us how we think (Brown 1970). In that word two entire complex and important fields, the psychological and the social, have been merged into one small term.

Perhaps in psychiatry we are living out Piaget's theories of genetic epistemology (Piaget 1950), which stated that the development of cognitive abilities in a child and the development of cognitive abilities in a society follow similar paths. Piaget described, for example, the situation in which the child was confronted with two glasses of equal height, one having a diameter twice that of the other. The thinner glass was filled with water, which was then poured into the wider glass. The level, of course, went much lower in the second glass and the child was asked whether it was still the same amount of water. Up to a certain stage of development, the child would say "no, there is less water in the wider glass" (because the level is lower). If the water was poured back into the thinner glass, the child would say "now there's more water." Piaget (1941) viewed the problem as the child's not having learned yet to attend to more than one dimension, in this case a focus on height. Piaget considered that simultaneous attention to height and diameter would be required for the child to attain the notion of volume and be able to understand the constancy of the volume of water, of matter.

By moving back and forth from one single emphasis to another in psychiatry, we may be preventing ourselves in a similar way from making optimal progress in developing essential concepts. We would deny it, just as psychoanalysts often did in the past. But our current situation, as with many social phenomena such as racism, may get part of its power from the difficulty in noticing what is happening when one is in its midst.

Now it seems, with impressive and increasing sophistication in the neurosciences, we are leaving patient description far behind. Although the rise of descriptive psychiatry and classification has been a boon to applying the neurosciences to mental illness, as the neurosciences have progressed to far more complex and dynamic understandings, the tendency to perseverate in our descriptive psychiatry and not to demand that it move along as well may be severely inhibiting our efforts. Through advances in the neurosciences we now recognize numerous transmitter systems, complex structural functional correlates in the brain, and complex changes over time such as lag periods, sequential alterations in brain structure and function, and feedback loops. Such complex mechanisms on one side of the equation are then compared to supposedly stable symptom-based diagnostic categories, static lumps, on the other.

Diagnostic Fit

If one focuses more carefully on the clinical description side of the equation, the psychological side of the field, it seems likely that the phenomenology of severe mental illness is quite different from, or at least quite inadequately covered by, many of our current diagnostic notions. The dynamic biologies are anchored to static, simplistic, descriptive notions rather than to the complexity, depth, and dynamism that appear more adequately to describe the real nature of functioning in patients with psychiatric disorders.

Even the notion of discrete diagnostic categories can be questioned. Clinicians frequently complain about the many patients who do not fit neatly into diagnostic groups. Many biological studies suggest that some findings, whether of brain structure, physiologic mechanisms, genetics, or psychopharmacologic action, transcend diagnostic categories to characterize, for example, all patients with psychosis whether the diagnosis is schizophrenia, bipolar disorder, or schizoaffective disorder (e.g., Wexler 1992). There is no reason to discount these findings and impressions merely because our diagnostic concepts do not match them.

In fact, as has been suggested, current diagnostic concepts may be only rough approximations of the complexities and diversities of clinical reality. In one report, for example (Strauss et al. 1979), a multivariate statistical approach was used to explore the actual distribution of patients' symptoms and syndromes in relation to diagnostic categories. Symptom ratings for a group of "archetypal patients" were fabricated to fit diagnostic categories. The data from these ratings were analyzed with a biplot algorithm, a statistical procedure somewhat like principal components analysis. Results demonstrated that the biplot procedure could reproduce clearly the diagnostic categories of the archetypal, fabricated patients. Symptom ratings from real patients, made on an epidemiologically representative sample of first hospital admissions for psychiatric disorder, were then analyzed with the biplot. Some of the symptom clusters were approximated by the real patients, but the patients themselves did not cluster neatly at all. Rather the patient distribution reflected a heterogeneous range of symptom combinations. These findings suggested that although diagnostic concepts were somewhat reflected in the correlations among symptoms, individual patients actually demonstrated a wide range of symptom combinations. It may be that the field of psychiatry, as though following the gestalt psychology notion of "good form" (Kohler 1933), has created stereotyped diagnostic clusters from poorly fitting data primarily to generate clear concepts.

If the processes involved in psychiatric disorder actually reflect continua and diversity rather than neat categories, then biological findings, including responses to pharmacologic agents that transcend diagnostic categories, may not be mere curiosities to be de-emphasized and ignored. Rather they may be trying to tell us something about the realities of biological phenomena in real psychiatric disorder.

Prognosis

An analogous situation to the problem of poorly fitting symptom-based diagnoses may also exist for the supposed prognostic validity of psychiatric disorders. Kraepelin's (1899/1904) notion of dementia praecox (forerunner to the concept of schizophrenia) included four different symptom group subtypes. He viewed these as reflecting one pathologic process, largely because of his belief that people with these various syndromes almost invariably had a downhill course. Kraepelin was building on Sydenham's (1676/1942) notion of the natural history of a disorder, which could be stated in modern terms as "diagnosis is prognosis." This is the extremely important although simple notion that if a diagnostic category is valid, it will define a process, and that process will have longitudinal integrity. This notion is potentially a very powerful one when it is accurate. However, research (e.g., Harding et al. 1987; McGlashan and Carpenter 1988; Strauss and Carpenter 1972) has shown that the prognosis of schizophrenia is not homogeneous.

There is also considerable evidence to show that not one but many aspects of outcome exist, aspects such as social relations functioning, symptom severity, occupational functioning, and need for hospitalization, and that different variables are the most powerful predictors for each of these various aspects of outcome (Strauss and Carpenter 1974). On the basis of such findings we suggested that the course of disorder is not a homogeneous process but rather is constituted of many systems, each of which has its own set of intercorrelated variables, and that these systems are open and linked in that they also influence each other. It was on the basis of this open-linked systems view that multiaxial diagnosis was originally recommended for DSM-III (American Psychiatric Association 1980; Strauss 1975; Williams 1985).

When the details of symptom and prognostic characteristics were considered together, still another concept emerged that was not suggested by diagnostic categories. J. Hughlings Jackson's notion of positive and negative symptoms was revived (Strauss et al. 1974). This distinction has been shown to be of considerable value in attempting to isolate biological processes.

A Reconsideration of Diagnostic Concepts

What this brief review has identified, then, is that systematic, careful patient description may lead to reconsideration of basic diagnostic concepts. Findings suggest that current categories may have been adequate to begin the bootstrapping process of understanding disorder, but that such categories may reflect simplistic, static notions that relate only very approximately to the core processes involved in psychopathology. Careful observation suggests that symptom subgroups, as in the negative/positive symptom distinction, may have more biological reality than at least certain diagnostic categories, that there may be continua where we have assumed discrete diseases, and that there are multiple interacting areas of functioning. All of these notions have been accepted by the field of psychiatry in one way or another even as it has attempted to maintain the hegemony of the major diagnostic categories.

But what happens with current diagnostic concepts if we attempt to follow the lead of careful systematic observation still further? What happens is that more processes begin to be suggested, complex processes that, although considered crucial by pioneers of modern psychiatry such as Kraepelin, Bleuler, and Freud, are now all but ignored. It is as though, pursuing the notion of the importance of measurement, we have assumed the false syllogism "measurement is important; some things cannot be readily measured; therefore those things are of no importance." But if there are phenomena that have been difficult to measure that may reflect core processes, and if we refuse to attend to these phenomena, then biology is going to be severely handicapped in finding biological connections to psychopathologic mechanisms.

An example of one complex phenomenon that has been relatively ignored recently is the "will." Kraepelin (1899/1904) and Bleuler (1911/1950) both noted that one of the key characteristics of dementia praecox or schizophrenia was the failure of the person's will, the loss of goal-directed activity. It is extremely difficult, of course, to measure the will—not nearly as easy as it is to assess the response to the question "Do you hear voices?" Perhaps for that reason we may have agreed implicitly not to notice the whole goal-directed aspect of human functioning in much of psychiatry in recent years. In our own work, for example, in a series of follow-along studies of people with severe mental disorders (Strauss et al. 1985), we reinterview subjects periodically over a 3-year period. The interviewers are investigators in the study, all of whom have clinical as well as research experience. Because we conduct repeated interviews with the same subjects, the subjects get to know the interviewers and begin to feel free to talk about things, sometimes things that the interviewers do not ask about. Thus one subject, after several interviews in which we inquired about the effects of treatment, work, and social relationships on her symptoms, asked why we never inquired about what she did to help herself. The answer was simple enough—it had never occurred to us.

Subsequently we systematically inquired into this specific aspect of will, or goal-directed behavior, and found that most patients in our study in fact do a great number of things to help control their symptoms (Breier and Strauss 1983). Different people, even within the same diagnostic categories, do different things. Thus, for example, some people with schizophrenia appear to help control their voices by keeping busy; others find that just the opposite, withdrawing, seems to work. Although it is difficult methodologically to demonstrate whether these efforts are effective, these kinds of reports are so common that it would be dangerous to assume without further evidence that they are inaccurate or irrelevant. It seems at least as likely that there are various psychological and neurophysiological configurations in these people, configurations that do not necessarily conform to diagnostic categories and that allow particular behaviors to have the impact of lessening hallucinatory experiences.

Such considerations of people's goal-oriented efforts to control their symptoms are really only the beginning of lifting the lid off Pandora's box. Recognizing that the will might be important in severe mental disorders throws us into the methodologically difficult areas of intentionality, teleology, sense of self, and identity. All of these are so heavily burdened with theoretical superstructures as well as methodological difficulties that it is little wonder that many in the field have tried to avoid them entirely. Nevertheless, with open and detailed observation these areas keep intruding themselves so much that perhaps the worst thing we can do from a scientific point of view is to pretend that they are not there (Strauss 1989b). What begins to appear, then, if one sees people with mental disorders in a setting that does not discourage them from describing diverse aspects of their experience, is that descriptive psychiatry starts to become more complex and more dynamic.

The Course of Disorder

In our work, we have become increasingly interested in course of disorder, in addition to outcome. Once one recognizes the heterogeneity of outcomes that have been demonstrated, the next reasonable question is, What are the processes by which different outcomes evolve? Again, if Sydenham and Kraepelin and the many others who have attended to longitudinal processes (including Freud and Piaget) are correct, presumably these processes have important psychological, biological, and social components and provide keys to basic mechanisms.

To pursue an inquiry into course rather than outcome alone, we started carrying out the repeated assessments of patients noted above (Strauss et al. 1985). This was done in spite of warnings (all justified) about the statistical problems that such repeated measurements raise. But it seemed better to follow this path than to assume it was possible to get an adequate notion of processes in the course of disorder by making measurements at only two points in time. In fact, traditional outcome studies, including our own (e.g., Strauss and Carpenter 1974), using such two-point measures (or even using only two-point analyses when three or more points of data were collected) had often suggested that course of disorder, whether ending in improvement or deterioration, followed essentially a straight line. Once we began charting course with repeated measures, however, we found that what appears to be the one consistent finding is that no patient's course follows a straight line (Strauss et al. 1985). This finding raised the further question of whether variations from straight lines were merely noise in the measurement process or a signal indicating some underlying psychobiosocial process.

The research logistics and methodology for answering this question definitively are problematic. But observation, combined with patients' reports of the quality of their experiences, suggests that these nonlinear patterns in course may reflect relatively specific phases of disorder. Some of these phases may have a purpose and a mechanism, just as do phases of bacterial growth, human physical development, and human intellectual development.

For example, one phase in the course of psychiatric disorder that has been suggested is "woodshedding" (Strauss 1989a). Often after a patient has recovered slightly from a severe decompensation, there is a plateau of functioning. At this point, clinicians, patients, and family members often wonder if the person is burning out or becoming chronic, or if in some way the treatment is failing. Having observed the experiences of many patients going through this period, there is now reason to hypothesize that in many instances at least, such patients are experiencing a woodshedding phase. This is a period during which the patient is actually accumulating strengths, including self-esteem and abilities to function socially, but these changes are occurring at levels too low to permit measurement by general scales. When asked, after such a phase has ended, many patients state spontaneously that of course they needed to go through that kind of period. As one subject told us who had just started working after several years being unemployed, it was like baking a cake. You can get flour, but you still can't make a cake; then you get the butter and you still can't make a cake; but when you get everything there, then you can make the cake. Following such a woodshedding phase, patients frequently take a job, move out of the parental household, or in other ways make a major step forward. The word "woodshedding" was suggested by Lieberman (Strauss et al. 1985) from the use of the term by jazz musicians. When these musicians attempt to develop a new style, rather than performing in public where their mistakes are all too obvious and disconcerting, they retreat to the isolation of the "woodshed" until the more obvious problems have been worked out.

If such phases of disorder do exist, they have major implications for the underlying psychological and biological mechanisms that may be involved in the processes of disorder and improvement. For example, patients frequently seem to pass through phases knowingly (existence of the woodshedding phase was first suggested by a patient who, after hospitalization, returned to the parental home because she said she needed a period of "unconditional love"). This and other observations from our work suggest that the course of disorder may be influenced by self-regulatory processes and that control theory, postulating the regulation of a system by its own monitoring and control mechanisms, including processes of perception, interpretation (meaning), and action, is involved. Viewed from this perspective, common notions such as "noncompliance" with medication may indeed reflect negativism or laziness as is sometimes suggested, but may also represent the utilization of a self-regulatory process by the person with the disorder. There may, for example, be a time in the course of illness when a particular medication may in fact seem inappropriate for the needs at that time. A person whose work helps him or her control symptoms, but for whom medication causes lethargy or stiffness that makes working impossible, is faced with a complex regulatory problem that goes far beyond "compliance."

Developmental Aspects

If processes involving the will and self-regulation are central to understanding psychiatric disorder and its course, then one more aspect of course also needs to be considered. The self that is being regulated exists over time, a time that both precedes and follows the actual occurrence of measurable disorder. Since selves have at least some degree of continuity, a notion of development must be considered in understanding these processes. Unfortunately, development is another concept in psychiatry heavily burdened with theory, thus driving away many empiricists from even considering it in regard to severe mental disorder. Nevertheless, if we are to understand processes that may underlie psychopathology and course, it may be foolhardy to avoid this area.

For example, one subject in our study described some "bizarre behavior" (as we originally rated it) that occurred early in the course of her illness, when she was about 32 years old. By the time of our first research interview about 6 years later, she had been given the DSM-III diagnosis of schizoaffective disorder. After her first psychotic episode and hospitalization, she had been discharged and then began hitchhiking, certainly a dangerous practice for her, and one that was considered by others and ourselves as "bizarre behavior." At our follow-up research interview 2 years after our initial assessment, this woman, who has not had any intensive psychodynamic treatment and has had a limited education, volunteered that, looking back at the time when she got sick, she felt that she had been very much tied to her mother's apron strings. She further volunteered that when she was hitchhiking it was the first time she had been away from home, and although sometimes she was exploited, in some instances she met people who really seemed to value her and take her seriously as a person.

Thus this piece of "bizarre behavior" was certainly unwise, but from a developmental perspective may have been not just bizarre but an effort to become autonomous and develop self-esteem. Like a tree trying to grow through a concrete slab, this woman may have been trying to grow, even though in a potentially distorted and self-defeating way. The meanings of such behavior in a developmental context may be crucial. Ignoring such meanings (e.g., by viewing the behavior only as bizarre), as difficult as they are to study systematically, may be antiscientific and may defeat efforts to understand underlying psychological, biological, and social mechanisms.

Developmental meanings can have a major role in other aspects of disorder as well, even in such basic symptoms as hallucinations. There are many examples of hallucinatory content and context reflecting major developmental issues for a patient. One of our subjects reported that her voices got worse whenever she tried to return to college. This worsening seemed closely related to her problems in leaving her lower-class ethnic background. One does not need to assume that developmental meanings are the only relevant aspects of such symptoms, but it is crucial to question the practice of looking only at the superficial aspects of symptoms while systematically ignoring possible implications of their developmental meaning. It may after all be the psychology and biology of meaning rather than the psychology and biology of auditory experience that is the crucial process involved in such symptoms.

Conclusions

Proceeding beyond descriptive classification that is limited to relatively superficial observations to more careful longitudinal observation of subjects has led to considering issues of will, self-regulation, meaning, and developmental contexts. Patients report behaviors and feelings reflecting these issues as readily as they report, for example, hearing voices and belief in delusional ideas, as long as we let them know that we are interested and allow them to get to know us well enough so that they feel free to mention the deeper and more complex aspects of their experience. This shift in scope of what we allow ourselves to observe leads to a shift from more static notions of disorder to the consideration of various areas of function, to concepts like will and phases of change.

In addition, a relatively open and intensive approach to descriptive psychiatry suggests that single diagnostic interviews, although useful for some purposes, may in fact preclude adequate description. It is obvious that just because we see people only once or twice for a diagnostic assessment or outcome evaluation or categorize them only once does not mean that there is not more happening. In descriptive psychiatry it is not adequate to assume that if we do not see it, it does not exist, that out of our sight is necessarily out of someone else's mind.

The Decade of the Brain may lead to many advances in the neurosciences and to understanding aspects of psychiatric disorder. But having a decade of integration of biological, psychological, and social aspects of psychiatry would be better. While investigators in the neurosciences are studying the intricate dynamics of brain functioning, clinicians and researchers in descriptive psychiatry are generally dealing with static diagnostic categories, limiting observations to the most superficial of the data potentially available. In any science, one does not carry out calculations to decimal points beyond the error of measurement. In psychiatry, the sophistication of biological psychiatry has far outstripped the sophistication of our research observations of patients. The Decade of the Brain for psychiatry may be only as successful as the adequacy of our clinical assessment will allow. Psychiatry is a psychobiosocial field, but parts of the field focusing on psychological and social factors need to progress. We need to develop a dynamic descriptive psychiatry to complement the dynamic models of modern neuroscience.

References

American Psychiatric Association: Diagnostic and Statistical Manual of Mental Disorders, 3rd Edition. Washington, DC, American Psychiatric Association, 1980

Bleuler E: Dementia praecox or the group of schizophrenias (1911). Translated by Zinken J. New York, International Universities Press, 1950

Breier A, Strauss JS: Self-control in psychotic disorders. Arch Gen Psychiatry 40:1141–1145, 1983

Brown R: Psycholinguistics. New York, Free Press, 1970

Harding CM, Brooks GW, Ashikaga T, et al: The Vermont longitudinal study, II: long-term outcome of subjects who retrospectively met the DSM-III criteria for schizophrenia. Am J Psychiatry 144:727–735, 1987

Kohler W: Psychologische Probleme. Berlin, Springer, 1933

Kraepelin E: Dementia praecox and paraphrenia, in Textbook of Psychiatry, 1899, 6th German edition. Translated and edited by Defendorff AR. New York, Macmillan, 1904

McGlashan T, Carpenter WT Jr (eds): Long-term follow-up studies of schizophrenia (special issue). Schizophrenia Bulletin 14(4), 1988

Piaget J: Introduction a l'Epistemologie Genetique. Paris, Presses Universitaires de France, 1950

Piaget J, Inhelder B: Le Developpement Desquantiter Chez l'Enfant. Neuchâtel, Switzerland, Delachaux et Niestle, 1941

Rutter M: Stress, coping and development: some issues and some questions. J Child Psychol Psychiatry 22:323–356, 1981

Strauss JS: A comprehensive approach to psychiatric diagnosis. Am J Psychiatry 132:1193–1197, 1975

Strauss JS: Mediating processes in schizophrenia: towards a new dynamic psychiatry. Br J Psychiatry 155:22–28, 1989a

Strauss JS: Subjective experiences of schizophrenia: towards a new dynamic psychiatry. Schizophr Bull 15:179–187, 1989b

Strauss JS, Carpenter WT Jr: Prediction of outcome in schizophrenia, I: characteristics of outcome. Arch Gen Psychiatry 27:739–746, 1972

Strauss JS, Carpenter WT Jr: Prediction of outcome in schizophrenia, II: relationships between predictor and outcome variables. Arch Gen Psychiatry 31:37–42, 1974

Strauss JS, Carpenter WT Jr: The key clinical dimensions in the functional psychoses, in Biology of the Major Psychoses. Edited by Freedman DX. New York, Raven, 1975

Strauss JS, Carpenter WT Jr, Bartko JJ: Speculations on the processes that underlie schizophrenic symptoms. Schizophr Bull 11:61–70, 1974

Strauss JS, Gabriel RK, Kokes RF, et al: Do psychiatric patients fit their diagnoses? patterns of symptomatology as described with the biplot. J Nerv Ment Dis 167:105–113, 1979

Strauss JS, Hafez H, Lieberman P, et al: The course of psychiatric disorder, III: longitudinal principles. Am J Psychiatry 142:289–296, 1985

Sydenham T: On scarlet fever, from Observationes Medical circa Morborum Actuorum Historiam et Curationem (1676) (translated by Lathan RG, Medical Classics, 4(4), December 1939), in Clendening L: Source Book of Medical History. New York, Dover, 1942, pp 198–199

Wexler B: Beyond the Kraepelinian dichotomy. Biol Psychiatry 31:539–541, 1992

Williams JBW: The multiaxial system of DSM-III: where did it come from and where should it go? Arch Gen Psychiatry 42:175–186, 1985

Section II

The Phenomenology of Schizophrenia

The Phenomenology of Schizophrenia

◆

The term *phenomenology* has a variety of meanings in philosophy and in psychiatry. It derives from the Greek word *phenomenon,* which means "appearance." In classical philosophy a distinction was made between appearance and reality. Over time, *phenomenon* gradually came to mean "that which is externally observable." It had more or less this meaning in the work of Hegel, who wrote a major work on the phenomenology of mind. In the writings of Jaspers and Heidiger, it acquired the special meaning of "the externally observable which is used to perceive the inner experience." In the language of medical psychiatry, it evolved to mean externally observable signs and symptoms. In contemporary American psychiatric terminology, a distinction is made between the study of signs and symptoms of disease, which is referred to as phenomenology, and the study of disease classifications or categories, which is referred to as nosology. This section of the book explores phenomenology from the perspective of contemporary American psychiatry.

In its early stages, the study of phenomenology emphasized careful description of signs and symptoms. In Chapter 4, my colleagues and I summarize our work on phenomenology at the University of Iowa. The effort has involved the development of standardized measurement instruments, which provide reliable methods for identifying the severity of various signs and symptoms of serious mental illness. This approach to phenomenology belongs within the traditions of German descriptive psychiatry and British empirical psychiatry. However, contemporary phenomenology has moved beyond an attempt merely to define signs and symptoms carefully to an attempt to understand how signs and symptoms arise from their underlying neural mechanisms. The effort to link specific signs and symptoms to neural mechanisms is illustrated in Chapter 4, with a particular focus on negative symptoms and frontal lobe pathology.

A different approach to phenomenology is provided in Chapter 5, in which Dr. Ruben C. Gur and his colleagues describe the application of the techniques of neuropsychology to understand brain function in schizophrenia. In this case, the emphasis is on measuring mental behavior (i.e., psychometrics) rather than measuring signs and symptoms. That is, instead of evaluating hallucinations, delusions, or disorganized speech, and attempting to relate these aberrations in mental functioning to underlying neural mechanisms, these authors describe an effort to measure abstraction, memory, spatial skills, and other mental abilities, and to link deficits in these various areas to the presence of schizophrenia.

Chapter 6 provides yet another approach to phenomenology. Dr. Adrianne M. Reveley describes how the study of identical twins can be used to explore the clinical presentation of schizophrenia and to identify its underlying genetic and environmental mechanisms. Monozygotic twins provide a fascinating "natural laboratory," in that they share identical genetic material. Consequently, any differences that are noted in twins must be due to environmental influences, which are broadly defined to include anything that is nongenetic, such as prenatal influences (as indicated by birth weight), birth injuries, or infections early in life. Dr. Reveley summarizes work involving twin studies of schizophrenia and continues the effort to link the study of phenomenology to underlying neural mechanisms.

Chapter 4

The Neural Mechanisms of Mental Phenomena

Nancy C. Andreasen, M.D., Ph.D.
Victor W. Swayze III, M.D.
Michael Flaum, M.D.
Daniel S. O'Leary, Ph.D.
Randall Alliger, Ph.D.

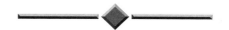

> The fact that there is only one word to refer to a thing does not mean that there is only one thing.
>
> Ludwig Wittgenstein

Identifying the neural mechanisms of mental phenomena has been a goal of clinician-scientists for more than a century. This topic has fascinated individuals as diverse as Freud and Kraepelin. Linking clinical symptoms to underlying brain mechanisms was the subject of one of Freud's early works, *Project for a Scientific Psychology* (Freud 1895/1966). Kraepelin's textbook on dementia prae-

This research was supported in part by NIMH Grants MH31593, MH40856, and MHCRC 43271; The Nellie Ball Trust Fund; Iowa State Bank and Trust Company, Trustee; and a Research Scientist Award, MH00625.

cox (1919) returns repeatedly to the issue of how the various symptoms of schizophrenia can be understood in terms of what is known about brain structure and function. Kraepelin clearly anticipated many of the ideas that are currently being explored by investigators attempting to understand the neural substrates of the symptoms of schizophrenia in the 1990s. At the turn of the century, prior to the description of the limbic system, Kraepelin wrote:

> If it should be confirmed that the disease attacks by preference the frontal areas of the brain, the central convolutions or the temporal lobes, this distribution would in a certain measure agree with our present views about the site of the psychic mechanisms which are principally injured by the disease. On various grounds it is easy to believe that the frontal cortex, which is specially well developed in man, stands in closer relation to his higher intellectual abilities, and these are the faculties which in our patients invariably suffer profound loss in contrast to memory acquired abilities. The manifold volitional and motor disorders, which extend partly to the harmonious working of the muscles, will make us think of finer disorders in the neighborhood of the precentral convolution. . . . On the other hand the peculiar speech disorders resembling sensory aphasia and the auditory hallucinations, which play such a large part, probably point to the temporal lobe being involved. (p. 19)

It is a fundamental given that the symptoms of an illness such as schizophrenia can be explained in terms of disruptions in normal brain activity. Symptoms such as hearing voices, intellectual emptiness, or garbled, disorganized speech must arise ultimately from an aberration in the functions of perception, processing, and production of information in the brains of people who are experiencing these symptoms. The past century has taught us a great deal about normal cognitive processes. Simpler systems such as visual perception have been mapped with increasing sophistication, and we are steadily learning more about other functions such as auditory processing, language perception and production, memory, and attention. When a patient with schizophrenia experiences a symptom such as an abnormal perception (i.e., an auditory hallucination), this is not produced by a "ghost in the machine" but rather by some type of abnormality in the brain systems that affect language perception and processing, ranging from the primary auditory cortex on through the complex interlinked circuits involved in monitoring and producing speech.

Despite this fundamental given, neither Freud, nor Kraepelin, nor

Kleist, nor Leonhard, nor the many others who followed them have as yet succeeded in explaining the symptoms of schizophrenia in terms of underlying brain functions. During this final decade of the 20th century, which has been officially declared the Decade of the Brain by Congress, achieving such an understanding is one of the major goals of the psychopathology of schizophrenia. As yet, we are not able to explain a single sign or symptom of schizophrenia on the basis of neural mechanisms. Nevertheless, this remains the long-term goal of a scientific psychopathology. The problems that investigators face during the 1990s are similar to those faced by early investigators. Although the hope of achieving this goal is a real one, the road toward it will be arduous.

Problems in Developing Models: Phenomenological Aspects

Despite recent advances in neuroscience, the illness that we call schizophrenia has not yielded itself easily to understanding because of problems on multiple fronts. One major front is the phenomenology of the illness. Some of the problems encountered in developing models to explain the psychopathology of schizophrenia are summarized in Table 4–1.

Although considerable progress has been made in clinical description through the development of a variety of structured interviews and rating scales, the definitions of the symptoms of schizophrenia are sometimes crude or unreliable (Andreasen and Flaum 1990). Some symptoms (e.g., positive formal thought disorder and negative symptoms such as affective blunting or avolition) have elicited particular concern about poor reliability. Rating scales developed since the 1980s have, however, made substantial advances in this area.

Table 4–1.   Problems in developing models: phenomenological aspects

- Crude and unreliable definition of symptoms
- Diversity of characteristic symptoms
- Evolution or modulation of symptoms over time
- Difficulties in studying symptoms independently of medication effects
- Probable inherent heterogeneity of schizophrenia

The diversity of the symptoms that characterize schizophrenia also presents major conceptual problems. Any model that attempts to explain symptoms on the basis of neural mechanisms must address this issue, which has several facets. First, schizophrenia is a polythetic illness, and there is no single defining feature for it. Thus, to be considered definitive, a model must be able to explain why some patients have hallucinations, disorganized speech, and affective blunting, whereas others have persecutory delusions, avolition, and anhedonia. A second facet of the problem is presented by the fact that the various symptoms of schizophrenia encompass multiple cognitive and behavioral domains. It is difficult to develop models that can explain how symptoms potentially involving so many different brain systems can co-occur within the same individual. Another facet of the problem arises because these diverse symptoms do not necessarily remain constant over time. Some patients with schizophrenia present initially with florid psychotic symptoms, which subsequently "burn out"; others show variability in phenomenology from one exacerbation to another. The effects of medication further complicate the evaluation of phenomenology. Its therapeutic effects may diminish the severity of positive symptoms, while its side effects may worsen the severity of negative symptoms. Removing patients from medication to evaluate the severity of psychopathology is difficult in many research settings, but it may be the only accurate way of determining the nature and severity of psychopathology in any given patient.

A final problem in assessing the phenomenology of schizophrenia and in developing neuropathological models to explain it is the probable inherent heterogeneity of schizophrenia itself. As Wittgenstein (1958) reminded us, just because there is only one word to refer to the disease "schizophrenia," we cannot infer that there is in fact only one disease. The clinical heterogeneity is one clue that suggests that the neuropathology and etiology are probably heterogeneous as well. There are also many other indicators. Research investigations of schizophrenia, no matter what the measure, are notoriously difficult to replicate. This difficulty in replication probably does not reflect on the quality of scientific methods being applied; rather, it suggests that investigators in different institutions may be looking at different samples from an inherently heterogeneous population. Another indicator of the heterogeneity of schizophrenia is the repeated observation that samples of patients diagnosed as having schizophrenia tend to have a much larger standard deviation than a control or comparison group on almost everything that has been measured; this large standard deviation is suggestive of true inherent diversity. Research studies on the etiology of schizophrenia also suggest diversity: although there is strong evidence for a genetic etiology from twin studies and other genetic techniques, family studies indicate that the base rate in first-degree relatives of index cases is relatively low, suggesting a rather weak genetic effect. Other approaches, such as studies of season of birth or rates of birth injury, suggest that environmental factors may also play a role in etiology. Potentially, schizophrenia may be a final common pathway much like mental retardation, with some patients having a prominently genetic disorder and other patients having a disorder with a strong environmental input; yet, at the clinical level, these two types of schizophrenia may be indistinguishable.

Problems in Developing Models: Neural Aspects

If the clinical side of the equation contains many terms, so does the neuroscience side. Some of the problems encountered in developing models to understand the psychopathology of schizophrenia, as seen from the perspective of neuroscience, are summarized in Table 4–2.

One fundamental aspect of the problem is the lack of animal models. Many of the symptoms of schizophrenia are disruptions of cognitive and behavioral functions that occur only in human beings, at least to a highly developed level. Since only human beings have language, animal models for formal thought disorder are not possible. Likewise, auditory hallucinations, which usually involve verbal content, cannot be modeled. Amphetamine-induced hypervigilance is a relatively weak model for the

---

Table 4–2.   Problems in developing models: neural aspects

- Inadequate animal models
- No clear neurological models
- Anatomical complexity
- Neurochemical complexity
- Functional complexity
- Difficulty in integrating information about structure and function
- Limitations in knowledge about structure and function of the human brain
- Need for in vivo as well as in vitro studies

---

complex aberrations in inferential thinking that characterize the delusional thinking of schizophrenic patients. The animal models used by pharmaceutical companies to test therapeutic efficacy of antipsychotics (e.g., catalepsy, stereotypy, rotatory behavior) are also weak models. The strongest animal models, which examine complex sequential planning and other cognitive functions, require the use of primates. Research of this type must necessarily be done in a relatively limited number of settings.

In addition to the lack of animal models, there are no clear neurological models for schizophrenia. Specific symptoms can be partially modeled, but in general their presentation is subtly different in neurological illnesses than in the psychiatric illness that we refer to as schizophrenia, suggesting that the mechanisms producing these symptoms may be different in some important way. For example, schizophrenic patients display poverty of speech, as do patients with Broca's aphasia, but schizophrenic patients lack the agrammatism and the subjective frustration displayed by patients with Broca's aphasia. Patients with Wernicke's aphasia speak in a garbled and disorganized manner that can be similar to the positive formal thought disorder of schizophrenia, but patients with schizophrenia typically show normal comprehension of the speech of others, whereas patients with Wernicke's aphasia do not. The masklike facies of patients with Parkinson's disease is similar to affective blunting in schizophrenia, but parkinsonian patients often do not experience a subjective sense of emotional emptiness or emotional withdrawal; this emotional emptiness or withdrawal may be an important part of affective blunting in schizophrenia. Although these examples suggest that language circuitry or dopamine projections may be important places to look in the effort to understand dysfunctions of language and affect in schizophrenia, they also suggest that investigators who do so should proceed with considerable caution and beware of oversimplifying.

Other problems in developing models to understand the neural substrates of mental phenomena arise from the great complexity of the human brain. This complexity exists at the level of anatomy, neurochemistry, and functional organization. The explosion in neuroscience has produced masses of information in all these domains, which certainly provides a growing and important knowledge base that can be used to understand neural aspects of schizophrenia; on the other hand, the knowledge base is growing so exponentially that it is difficult for a single investigator to achieve an adequate integration of all available information. Further, the knowledge base concerning the human brain still remains limited in comparison to knowledge about other animals, largely because of the inherent problems involved in studying the human brain (e.g., lack of postmortem tissue and difficulty in doing in vivo studies).

A Sequential Program for Studying the Phenomena of Mental Illness

When confronting problems that are highly complex, one useful coping strategy is to develop a sequential or serial approach to studying them. If all facets of the problem are attacked simultaneously, then efforts may become fragmented, disorganized, and ultimately even demoralized. Table 4–3 outlines a sequential program for studying the phenomena of mental illness. The program consists of three stages, each of which builds on earlier work.

Clinical description is the first stage. To examine the relationship between mental phenomena and neural mechanisms, one must have adequate techniques for assessing the phenomena. The first stage involves identifying which signs and symptoms are of interest. Approaches may vary, but our own bias is toward identifying a thorough and comprehensive list of phenomena that are assessed in a standardized manner. These phenomena are evaluated through an extensive structured interview, the Comprehensive Assessment of Symptoms and History (CASH) (Andreasen et al. 1992). Once a specific group of phenomena are identified, then techniques must be developed to assess them reliably, preferably evaluating both interrater and test-retest reliability. Whenever possible, both observational items and self-report items should be used.

The second stage involves assessment through standardized tests. At our present stage of development, these tend to draw on the techniques

---

Table 4–3.   Studying phenomena of mental illness: a sequential program

Clinical description.   The development of reliable methods to measure the phenomena in a clinical setting through observation and self-report

Neuropsychological and neurophysiological description.   The development of reliable methods to measure the cognitive and physical manifestations of the phenomena

Determination of mechanisms and causes.   The development of techniques for understanding the symptom in terms of brain structure and function

of neuropsychology and neurophysiology to provide relatively precise and reliable measurements of cognition and physiological function.

The third stage in this sequential program involves the use of techniques that provide a more direct method for assessing mechanisms and causes of the phenomena. The techniques of neuropsychology and neurophysiology are indirect measures, whereas techniques such as magnetic resonance imaging or positron-emission tomography (PET) permit investigators to study brain structure and function directly.

Clinical Assessment of the Symptoms of Schizophrenia

Because schizophrenia is so phenomenologically complex, another useful coping strategy is to simplify techniques for assessing clinical presentations so that they can be studied in an objective and quantitative way. One approach to simplifying the symptoms of schizophrenia that investigators have found to be of heuristic value is to divide them into positive and negative symptoms.

Table 4–4 lists positive and negative symptoms in a schematic format. Positive symptoms can be conceptualized as excesses or distortions of normal functions; negative symptoms are best conceptualized as decreases in or loss of normal functions.

Table 4–4.   Symptoms of schizophrenia

Positive Symptoms: Excessive or Distorted Function

Symptom	*Function disturbed*
Hallucinations	Perception
Delusions	Cognitive and inferential thinking
Positive formal thought disorder	Language
Bizarre behavior	Behavioral organization and control

Negative Symptoms: Loss or Diminution of Function

Symptom	*Function lost*
Alogia	Fluency of thought and speech
Affective blunting	Fluency of emotional expressiveness
Avolition	Volition and drive
Anhedonia	Emotional attachment and hedonic capacity
Attentional impairment	Attention

Although there is some controversy about which symptoms should be classified as positive or negative, an emerging consensus indicates that the following are probably positive symptoms: hallucinations, delusions, positive formal thought disorder, disorganized behavior, and inappropriate affect. Factor analytic studies have somewhat consistently suggested that these positive symptoms can be further subdivided into two factors. Delusions and hallucinations tend to be correlated with one another and to load on a psychoticism factor. Disorganized speech, disorganized behavior, and inappropriate affect are also correlated with one another and load on a separate factor (Andreasen and Grove 1986; Arndt et al. 1991; Bilder et al. 1985; Liddle 1987; McGorry et al. 1990a, 1990b). Table 4–5 shows a factor analysis completed by our group with the corresponding factor loadings for these various symptoms.

Negative symptoms, on the other hand, tend to be relatively tightly correlated with one another. Current consensus suggests that the following probably represent negative symptoms: alogia, affective blunting, avolition, anhedonia, and attentional impairment. Although the agreement on the first four is relatively solid, there is more controversy about attentional impairment, which in some studies has loaded with positive symptoms. In each case, however, these negative symptoms represent a diminution in cognitive and emotional capacities that are important aspects of daily living activities.

We have developed extensive standardized techniques for evaluating these positive and negative symptoms in our patients. This work has in-

Table 4–5. Varimax rotated factor loadings from the pooled covariance of the three studies ($N = 207$)

Factor	Study 1	Study 2	Study 3
Avolition	.82	.16	.01
Anhedonia	.81	−.01	.01
Affective flattening	.79	.07	.18
Alogia	.73	.46	.00
Attentional deficit	.72	.21	.16
Positive formal thought disorder	.07	.86	.12
Bizarre behavior	.22	.70	−.01
Delusions	−.03	.11	.83
Hallucinations	.22	−.02	.78

volved the development of two rating scales, the Scale for the Assessment of Negative Symptoms (SANS) and the Scale for the Assessment of Positive Symptoms (SAPS) (Andreasen 1982, 1983, 1984, 1985a, 1985b, 1989, 1990; Andreasen and Grove 1986; Andreasen and Olson 1982). In developing these scales, we stressed the selection of items that could be evaluated objectively whenever possible. This strategy was particularly important in developing techniques for assessing negative symptoms, which have tended to be de-emphasized until recently because they were thought to be unreliable.

Table 4–6 lists the items that are used to assess affective blunting, along with the reliability coefficients for each of these items. As the table indicates, a somewhat subjective concept has been objectified by asking the clinician to systematically examine and observe various objective components of the patient's behavior and emotional expression. The clinician is asked to assess eye contact, affective responsiveness, use of expressive gestures, and a variety of other details that are used by normal individuals to communicate their feelings and emotions to others. In general, good reliability is achieved for all of these items. In addition, having broken down affective blunting into its component parts through careful observation, the clinician is asked to make a global assessment of the severity of affective blunting. This global rating is also quite reliable. As

Table 4–6. Interrater reliability of the Scale for the Assessment of Negative Symptoms in three different cultural settings

	Intraclass r (weighted K)		
	Italy (Moscarelli et al. 1987)	Spain (Humbert et al. 1986)	Japan (Ohta et al. 1984)
Affective flattening			
Unchanging facial expression	.786	.930	.805
Decreased spontaneous movements	.782	.940	.728
Paucity of expressive gestures	.757	.886	.671
Poor eye contact	.873	.897	.676
Affective nonresponsivity	.714	.774	.641
Inappropriate affect	.774	.805	.294
Lack of vocal inflections	.827	.963	.720
Subjective rating of affective flattening		.831	.553
Global rating of affective flattening	.688	.844	.721
Subscale score		.926	

this approach indicates, breaking a subjective concept down into its objective components is an excellent technique for achieving good reliability, which has been documented in a variety of cultural settings (Humbert et al. 1986; Moscarelli et al. 1987; Ohta et al. 1984).

Similar levels of reliability have been achieved for the other items in the SANS and the SAPS. Table 4–7 summarizes the reliability coefficients of global ratings for the various SANS and SAPS items, indicating that they tend to be consistently high (Andreasen et al. 1992).

Negative Symptoms and the Prefrontal Cortex

Many different models may be developed to link specific symptoms, or groups of symptoms, to their neural substrates. One model, which our group at the University of Iowa has been exploring for a number of years, is a possible relationship between negative symptoms and a dysfunction in the prefrontal cortex. This possible relationship will be the focus of the remainder of this chapter, which will explore evidence that we have accumulated from a variety of different types of samples and experimental techniques to examine this possible association.

The prefrontal cortex is the largest single region in the human brain, constituting approximately one-third of the overall cortical area (Fuster 1989). The enormous elaboration of prefrontal regions and the specialization of left-hemisphere regions for verbal language functions are probably the major features that differentiate the human brain from the brains of other "lower" animals. The prefrontal cortex is a massive association region. Its connections are shown in Figure 4–1. As Figure 4–1 indicates, the prefrontal cortex is joined by reciprocal connections to all areas of the neocortex (temporal, parietal, and occipital) as well as limbic regions such as the cingulate gyrus and hippocampus. These direct connections prepare it to receive input in all sensory modalities (auditory, spatial, and visual), as well as from emotional and attentional centers; in turn, the prefrontal cortex can integrate information from these various modalities and can provide direct responses that have been modulated by the influence of all higher cortical functions. In addition, the prefrontal cortex receives ascending input from the anterior ventral and medial thalamic nuclei, which in turn receive input from various brain stem regions, as well as anterior and inferior temporal lobe regions. Its circuitry also connects it back to brain stem regions both directly and indi-

Table 4–7. Comprehensive Assessment of Symptoms and History reliability study: positive and negative symptoms

Symptoms (global ratings)	Current		First 2 years of illness		Much of time since onset		Worst ever	
	Interrater	Test-retest	Interrater	Test-retest	Interrater	Test-retest	Interrater	Test-retest
Positive symptoms								
Delusions	.76	.71	.74	.68	.64	.74	.83	.66
Hallucinations	.93	.65	.50	.62	.76	.65	.67	.48
Bizarre behavior	.62	.50	.28	.48	.30	.81	.82	.40
Positive formal thought disorder	.79	.62	.62	.41	.00	.52	.74	.73
Inappropriate affect	.61	.76	.71	.00	.67	.16	.68	.68
Sum of positive global ratings	*.86*	*.80*	*.64*	*.68*	*.71*	*.75*	*.82*	*.71*
Negative symptoms								
Affective flattening	.80	.76	.30	.13	.71	.55	.64	.40
Alogia	.66	.38	.73	.13	.45	.34	.63	.26
Apathy/avolition	.86	.67	.33	.00	.60	.54	.73	.37
Asociality/anhedonia	.81	.71	.18	.00	.53	.52	.62	.63
Attentional impairment	.67	.46	.59	.24	.27	.34	.81	.17
Sum of negative global ratings	*.86*	*.76*	*.63*	*.00*	*.73*	*.66*	*.88*	*.48*

rectly through thalamic way stations.

This schematic representation of prefrontal circuitry, which draws on the seminal descriptions of Fuster (1989), illustrates the inherent complexity of the prefrontal cortex. Not only must we worry about whether there is "one schizophrenia," but we must also worry about whether there is "one prefrontal cortex." The functions and specializations of the prefrontal cortex are still being mapped by many contemporary leaders in neuroscience. One traditional subdivision of the prefrontal cortex identifies three separate specialized regions: dorsolateral (subserving cognitive functions such as abstraction), orbital (subserving functions such as social judgment), and medial (governing activity and volition) (Cummings and Mendez 1984). Other theories of prefrontal function stress its role in monitoring and "understanding" the sequencing of events in

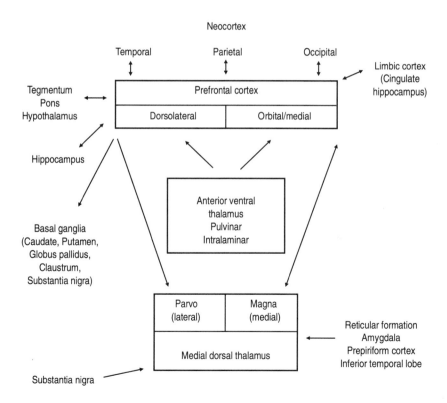

Figure 4–1. Connections of the prefrontal cortex.

time, prioritizing the importance of stimuli, referencing stimuli to internal representations, directing attention appropriately, and other "executive functions" (Fuster 1989; Goldman-Rakic 1984).

Our own work exploring the relationship between negative symptoms and the prefrontal cortex has focused on the evaluation of several different types of potentially informative populations and several different types of assessment strategy. One highly informative clinical population is a group of patients who were treated with prefrontal leukotomy in the state of Iowa during the late 1940s and early 1950s. As described in the next section of this chapter, we are conducting an extended follow-up study of these patients and assessing their social, cognitive, and neural function in a variety of ways. Because they have experienced relatively selective lesions to the prefrontal cortex, these subjects provide a "natural laboratory" for studying the neural substrates of frontal function and of negative symptoms. The second major clinical population that we have studied consists of patients with schizophrenia, who can be subdivided into groups with a high level of negative symptoms versus a low level of negative symptoms.

Both the leukotomized patients and the schizophrenic patients can be assessed clinically and evaluated in terms of severity of positive and negative symptoms, using the highly reliable rating instruments just described. In addition, they can be evaluated using the techniques of neuropsychology and neuroimaging, with an effort to determine interrelationships between negative symptoms, specific types of cognitive dysfunction, and specific types of neural dysfunction as assessed through measurement of regional cerebral blood flow. These studies are part of the large-scale program previously outlined that seeks to relate clinical phenomena to neural mechanisms in a sequential way. The remainder of this chapter will present some highlights from this work, which is still in progress.

Neural Substrates of Frontal Function: The Study of Leukotomized Patients

A large number of patients were treated with prefrontal leukotomy during the era before the development of neuroleptic drugs. Although the decision to use leukotomy on these patients appears to be a grave misjudgment when viewed retrospectively, and although the awarding of the Nobel prize to Moniz for the development of prefrontal leukotomy also appears to be a serious misjudgment in the history of science, in the context of the late 1940s these patients were considered to be hopeless and likely to be subjected to lifetime institutionalization. Nevertheless, it is still difficult to justify the widespread and uncritical use of leukotomy during the 1940s and 1950s.

Patients treated with this technique are now in their 60s and 70s. We have placed a high priority on attempting to identify as many of these patients as possible and to assess them comprehensively using clinical, neuropsychological, and neuroimaging techniques. We report here some preliminary data from a small sample of leukotomized patients identified and evaluated during the initial phases of the study. These patients are diagnostically heterogeneous, but the majority suffer from schizophrenia. Lesion size and site are variable, making cell sizes too small at present to seek specific correlations between lesion location and symptomatology or cognitive impairment.

The overall design of the study involves a clinical assessment that includes obtaining presurgical records to formulate a DSM-III-R (American Psychiatric Association 1987) diagnosis, completing the CASH on all subjects, documenting psychotropic medications used by patients, documenting total number of electroconvulsive therapy treatments received, and determining whether insulin coma was administered. In addition, we are attempting to document the various postoperative complications that have occurred, such as hemorrhage or coma, epileptic seizures, and urinary incontinence. Magnetic resonance is used to determine site and size of lesion. As this study matures, we will ultimately be able to examine interrelationships among types of symptomatology, size and site of lesion, and types of cognitive impairment. Location of lesion can be visualized through three-dimensional reconstruction. An example of this type of reconstruction is shown in Figure 4–2.

In our first analyses we compared 14 patients treated with leukotomy with 90 typical schizophrenic patients evaluated in our Mental Health Clinical Research Center who received a DSM-III (American Psychiatric Association 1980) diagnosis of schizophrenia. To examine the effects of leukotomy on positive and negative symptoms, we compared the severity of positive and negative symptoms in the two groups using the SANS and the SAPS. The results of these analyses are shown in Figures 4–3 and 4–4. As these figures indicate, the leukotomized patients had less severe symptoms as measured by both scales. The decreases in positive symptoms are not surprising. The lower negative symptoms are contrary, however, to a simple hypothesis postulating that leukotomy would worsen negative symptoms by damaging the higher executive centers located in the prefrontal cortex that mediate functions such as verbal fluency, volition, and attention. Thus the lower scores on negative symptoms in the leukotomized group were initially somewhat surprising. To examine the interrelationship between positive and negative symptoms and leukotomy in more detail, we conducted correlational analyses between the two symptom groups. The results of these analyses are shown in Table 4–8. As the table indicates, severity of positive and negative symptoms is not correlated in the nonleukotomized schizophrenic patients. Thus, in this group there is no relationship between severity of positive and negative symptoms. In the leukotomized patients, on the other hand, positive and negative symptoms are correlated.

What has the leukotomy done? These results suggest a preliminary theoretical explanation about the interrelationship between various

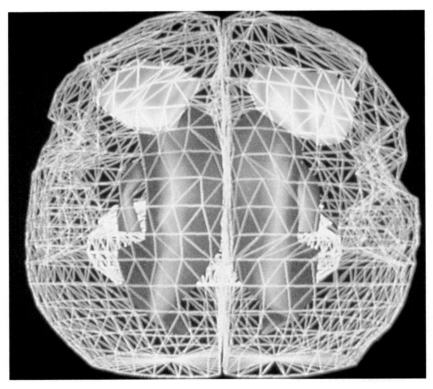

Figure 4–2. Three-dimensional reconstruction from a magnetic resonance scan showing lesion of leukotomized patient.

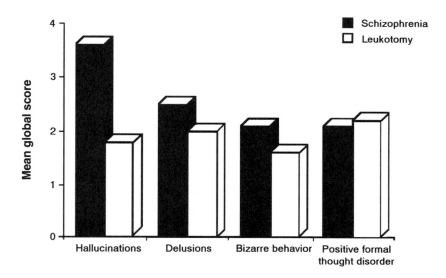

Figure 4–3.   Mean global scores on positive scales of the Scale for the Assessment of Positive Symptoms. The schizophrenic group has 90 subjects and the leukotomized group has 14 subjects.

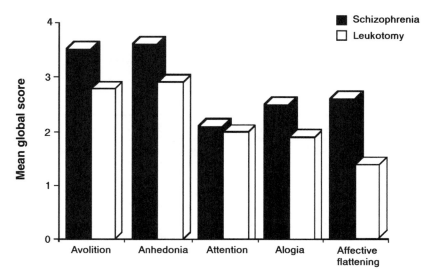

Figure 4–4.   Mean global scores on negative scales of the Scale for the Assessment of Negative Symptoms. The schizophrenic group has 90 subjects and the leukotomized group has 14 subjects.

brain centers in the production of positive and negative symptoms. As Figure 4–1 indicates, the prefrontal cortex has connections to many different brain centers that mediate a variety of functions. The leukotomy lesion may be presumed to have severed input to the prefrontal cortex from reticular, thalamic, and other subcortical "activating" centers, thereby increasing negative symptoms. On the other hand, it also has severed output from dorsolateral "executive" and integrative centers, releasing positive symptoms mediated through limbic and other subcortical regions. Thus the regions that might mediate positive and negative symptoms are "running free" without modulation in the leukotomized patients. Clearly, more work needs to be done to evaluate the pattern of symptoms in relation to size and site of lesion, but these preliminary findings are consistent with a plausible theory concerning the interaction between prefrontal cortical executive sites and subcortical limbic and other sites that may mediate positive symptoms. The results must be interpreted cautiously at present, however, for two reasons. First, the sample size is quite small. Second, the data are also consistent with the possibility that the "sickest" (i.e., most positive) patients were leukotomized; negative symptoms would then be superimposed on this preexisting positive substrate.

We have also completed preliminary evaluations of neuropsychological functioning in these leukotomized patients. We selected several from among a group of tasks that are commonly used to assess prefrontal cortical function. A comprehensive listing of putative "frontal" tasks is provided in Table 4–9. We selected three of these tasks to evaluate a relatively

---

Table 4–8.   Positive and negative symptoms in leukotomy patients

Nonleukotomized schizophrenic patients: positive and negative symptoms are uncorrelated

$r = .03$ for delusions and negative symptoms
$r = .14$ for hallucinations and negative symptoms
$r = .20$ for bizarre behavior and negative symptoms
$r = .23$ for positive formal thought disorder and negative symptoms

Leukotomized schizophrenic patients: positive and negative symptoms are correlated

$r = .74$ for delusions and negative symptoms
$r = .64$ for hallucinations and negative symptoms
$r = .56$ for bizarre behavior and negative symptoms
$r = .68$ for positive formal thought disorder and negative symptoms

broad range of prefrontal functions: the Wisconsin Card Sorting Test, the Stroop Color-Word Interference Test, and Trails B. The schizophrenic patients were further subdivided into those who had high negative symptoms and those who had low negative symptoms based on their SANS scores. The results of these analyses are shown in Figures 4–5, 4–6, and 4–7.

The leukotomized group performed much more poorly on the two

Table 4–9. Commonly used "frontal" tasks

Task	Function
Wisconsin Card Sorting Test	Simple abstraction, shifting response set
Continuous Performance Test	Sustained attention
Tower of London	Planning
Raven Progressive Matrices	High-level abstraction
Porteus Mazes	Planning
Stroop Color-Word Interference Test	Inhibiting interference
Trails B	Sustained attention

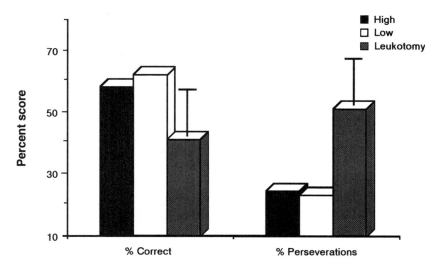

Figure 4–5. Wisconsin Card Sorting Test: percentage of correct responses and perseverations. The high-symptomatology group has 27 subjects, the low-symptomatology group has 39 subjects, and the leukotomized group has 10 subjects.

measures examined for the Wisconsin Card Sorting Test. They had a
smaller number of correct sortings and a substantially higher percentage
of negative responses. The leukotomized patients also were very impaired
on all components of the Stroop, including time to read a colored word,

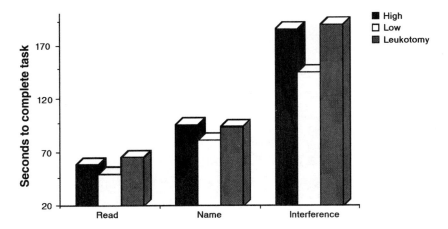

Figure 4–6. Results of the Stroop Color-Word Interference Test: time to read
a colored word, name a colored patch, and name the color in which the word
is printed.

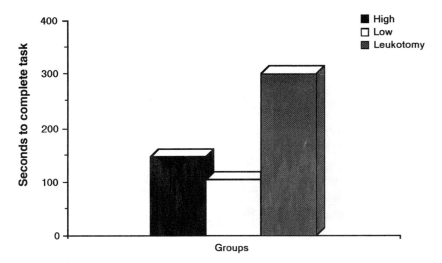

Figure 4–7. Trail Making Test time score. The high-symptomatology group
has 29 subjects, the low-symptomatology group has 43 subjects, and the
leukotomized group has 8 subjects.

to name a colored patch, and to name the color in which the word is printed. Finally, they also performed poorly on the Trail Making Test, taking substantially longer to complete the task. No striking differences were observed between the two schizophrenic groups on any of these tests. From this neuropsychological assessment, we can see that leukotomized patients have difficulty sustaining attention and performing high-level cognitive processing tasks that tap into the capacity to adapt to change and to inhibit interference. These findings are consistent with the hypothesis that the prefrontal cortex is responsible for monitoring and modulating multimodal input from a variety of brain regions and uses this information to integrate decision making during the process of task performance. Disconnection of prefrontal circuitry impairs these complex processes.

Insights From Functional Neuroimaging

Functional neuroimaging provides an alternative technique for exploring interrelationships between symptomatology and dysfunctions in specific brain regions. The pioneering work of Kety et al. (1948) led to the development of models for the measurement of cerebral blood flow and metabolism. Since that early work, applications have evolved that now permit visualization and measurement of brain physiology at a relatively high level of specificity. The major imaging modalities that are currently in use include single photon emission computed tomography (SPECT) and PET. SPECT permits the measurement of cerebral blood flow, using tracers such as [133]xenon, [123]IMP, and Tc-HMPAO. PET employs fluorodeoxyglucose to measure metabolism and ^{15}O-water to measure cerebral blood flow. Both of these techniques have been applied to address the "hypofrontality" issue in schizophrenia.

The earliest study was completed by Ingvar and Franzen (1974), who reported decreased perfusion in prefrontal cortex (as compared with that in occipital regions) in a small number of schizophrenic patients, who were compared with a control group. Since that time, a substantial literature has developed, which is summarized in Tables 4–10 and 4–11. As the tables indicate, the majority of the SPECT studies suggest that schizophrenic patients as a group have decreased cerebral blood flow both in the baseline state and when given a cognitive challenge. The PET studies are more evenly divided, but a substantial number of them also support the "hypofrontality hypothesis."

Table 4–10. Controlled cortical probe and SPECT studies evaluating frontal metabolism in schizophrenia

Study	Sample size	Test conditions	Medication status	Metabolic tracer	Results
Kety et al. 1948	22	Resting, sensory status not specified	No antipsychotics; other medication not specified	Nitrous oxide inhalation	No significant difference noted in schizophrenic patients vs. controls. (Only total cerebral blood flow measurement possible.)
Ingvar and Franzen 1974; Franzen and Ingvar 1975a, 1975b	31	Resting in quiet room with eyes blindfolded. Older psychotic group had simple picture test. Low-psychotic group had Raven's Progressive Matrices. Ten controls tested with auditory digit-span-backward test; 9 with Raven's Matrices	30/31 on variable dosages of anti-psychotics; all patients and controls pre-medicated with 200 mg pheno-barbital and 0.75 mg atropine	Intracarotid ^{133}Xe; 32 probes/left hemisphere only	*At rest:* No significant differences in frontal flow rates between schizophrenic patients and alco-holic controls. Postcentral flow significantly greater in older highly psychotic group than in alcoholic controls. Ratio of frontal to postcentral blood flow significantly less in schizophrenic patients than in alcoholic controls, thus "relative hypofrontality." *With cognitive activation:* Older high-psychotic group showed significantly less frontal flow response than alcoholic controls. (Note that two different cognitive tasks were used.) Trend for lower flow response was found in low-psychotic group compared with controls (for identical testing procedure, differences not significant).
Mathew et al. 1981	6	Resting, sensory status not specified	All off medication × 1 week	^{133}Xe inhalation; 16 probes/both hemispheres	Lower mean rCBF value for gray matter in schizophrenic patients vs. controls significant only for right hemisphere. No relative hypo-frontality reported.

Study	N	Condition	Medication	Method	Findings
Mathew et al. 1982	23	Resting, sensory status not specified	13 medicated, 9 off medication × 1 week, 1 unknown	^{133}Xe inhalation; 16 probes/both hemispheres	Mean blood flow in both hemispheres and in most brain regions studied was significantly lower in schizophrenic patients vs. controls. No relative hypofrontality reported.
Ariel et al. 1983	29	Resting, sensory status not specified	22 medicated	^{133}Xe inhalation; 16 probes/both hemispheres	Relative hypofrontality in left hemisphere of schizophrenic patients.
Gur et al. 1983	15	Resting, eyes open; verbal analogy test and spatial task	All medicated	^{133}Xe inhalation; 16 probes/both hemispheres	*At rest:* Increased frontal flow in both schizophrenic patients and controls. *With cognitive activation:* Schizophrenic patients had significantly less change in left-hemispheric flow for verbal analogy test than controls but a greater left-hemispheric increase for the spatial task.
Devous et al. 1985	34	Resting	All off medication × 7 days	^{133}Xe inhalation with SPECT	Hypofrontality noted.
Devous et al. 1985	19	Activation with WCS	All off medication × 7 days	^{133}Xe inhalation with SPECT	Decreased frontal flow during activation relative to resting state in schizophrenic patients.
Gur et al. 1985	19	Resting, eyes open, ears unoccluded; activation with verbal analogy test and spatial task	5 off medication × 1 year, 3 off medication × 2 months, 8 off medication × 7 days, 3 drug naive	^{133}Xe inhalation; 16 probes/both hemispheres	No hypofrontality noted.

(continued)

Table 4-10. Controlled cortical probe and SPECT studies evaluating frontal metabolism in schizophrenia *(continued)*

Study	Sample size	Test conditions	Medication status	Metabolic tracer	Results
Kurachi et al. 1985	16	Resting, eyes closed	All on medication	^{133}Xe inhalation; 16 probes/both hemispheres	Relative hypofrontality noted.
Warkentin et al. 1985	16	Resting, eyes covered (rCBF measured on admission; at 1, 2, and 4 weeks; and at discharge)	Not specified	^{133}Xe inhalation; 32 probes/both hemispheres	No significant relative hypofrontality on admission. Right frontal flow significantly decreased with medication.
Berman et al. 1986	24	Resting, eyes closed; activation with WCS and number matching task	All on medication	^{133}Xe inhalation; 32 probes/both hemispheres	Relative decreased prefrontal flow noted at rest. Neither absolute nor relative prefrontal flow noted with number matching. Relative prefrontal flow decreased significantly during WCS.
Berman et al. 1986	18	Two visual continuous performance tasks	All off medication × 4 weeks	^{133}Xe inhalation; 32 probes/both hemispheres	No differences in frontal activation noted with either task in patients vs. controls.

Study	N	Condition	Medication	Method	Findings
Chabrol et al. 1986	10	Resting, sensory status not specified	All drug naive	^{133}Xe inhalation; 32 probes/both hemispheres	Relative hypofrontality.
Guenther et al. 1986	16	Resting, sensory status not specified; motor activation dominant of right hand	12 drug naive, 4 drug washout × 1 week	^{133}Xe inhalation with SPECT	
Weinberger et al. 1986	20	Resting, eyes closed; activation with WCS and number matching task	All off medication 4–6 weeks	^{133}Xe inhalation; 32 probes/both hemispheres	Relative decreased prefrontal flow noted at rest. Neither absolute nor relative prefrontal flow noted with number matching. Relative prefrontal flow decreased significantly during WCS.
Geraud et al. 1987	51	Resting, eyes closed	13 not treated, 29 on neuroleptics, 9 washed off oral medication × 15 days and depot medication × 45 days	^{133}Xe inhalation; 32 probes/both hemispheres	Relative hypofrontality noted.
Berman et al. 1988	24	Resting, eyes closed; activation with Raven's Progressive Matrices and symbols matching task	All off medication > 4 weeks	^{133}Xe inhalation; 32 probes/both hemispheres	No hypofrontality noted.

(continued)

Table 4–10. Controlled cortical probe and SPECT studies evaluating frontal metabolism in schizophrenia *(continued)*

Study	Sample size	Test conditions	Medication status	Metabolic tracer	Results
Dousse et al. 1988	27	Resting, eyes closed	12 on medication < 10 days, 12 on medication 11–60 days, 3 drug naive	^{133}Xe intravenous; 26 probes/both hemispheres	No hypofrontality noted.
Mathew et al. 1988	108	Resting, sensory status not specified	46 off medication × 2 weeks, 62 medicated	^{133}Xe inhalation; 32 probes/both hemispheres	Relative hypofrontality noted.
Weinberger et al. 1988	16	Resting, eyes closed; activation with WCS and number matching task	All off medication at least 4 weeks	^{133}Xe inhalation; 32 probes/both hemispheres	At-rest data not reported. Neither absolute nor relative prefrontal flow noted with number matching. Relative prefrontal flow decreased significantly during WCS.
Bajc et al. 1989	28	Resting, sensory status not specified	20 medicated < 2 weeks, 8 medicated long-term	Tc99m-HMPAO SPECT	No hypofrontality noted.
Cohen et al. 1989	10	Resting, eyes open	All medicated long-term	Iodine-123 IMP SPECT	No hypofrontality noted.
Erbas et al. 1990	20	Resting, eyes closed	All medicated	Tc99m-HMPAO SPECT	Lower frontal hypofrontality noted.

	N	Condition	Task	Method	Findings
Paulman et al. 1990	40	20 medicated, 20 off medication 7–14 days	Resting, eyes open	^{133}Xe inhalation with SPECT	Relative hypofrontality noted.
Sagawa et al. 1990	53	All medicated	Resting, eyes closed	^{133}Xe inhalation with SPECT	Hypofrontality noted.
Warkentin et al. 1990	17	7 medicated, 6 off medication 3–12 months, 4 drug naive	Resting, eyes closed (rCBF measured on admission at 1 week, and at discharge in subgroup of 10 unmedicated patients)	^{133}Xe inhalation; 32 probes/both hemispheres	No hypofrontality noted on admission. Significant left-hemisphere hypofrontality noted between 1 week and discharge.
Wood and Flowers 1990	18	All off medication > 10 days	Activation with two trials of auditory Probe Recognition Memory task, eyes closed	^{133}Xe inhalation; 16 probes/both hemispheres	Relative hypofrontality as a result of greater anxiety on second recognition trial after presumed habituation.

Note. rCBF = regional cerebral blood flow. HMPAO = hexamethylpropylene amine oxime. WCS = Wisconsin Card Sorting Test.

Table 4–11. Controlled PET studies evaluating frontal metabolism in schizophrenia

Study	Schizophrenic sample size	Test conditions	Medication status	Metabolic tracer	Results
Buchsbaum et al. 1982	8	Resting, eyes closed	Off > 2 weeks	^{18}F-deoxyglucose	Reduced relative prefrontal glucose metabolism
Sheppard et al. 1983	12	Resting, eyes closed, open room	6 drug naive, 4 1–4 doses, 2 off 7 days	^{15}O	No difference in frontal ratio analysis
Buchsbaum et al. 1984	16	Somatosensory stimulation, eyes closed	Off > 2 weeks	^{18}F-deoxyglucose	Reduced relative prefrontal glucose metabolism
Farkas et al. 1984	11	Resting, eyes open, open room	6/13 medicated	^{18}F-deoxyglucose	Reduced relative prefrontal glucose metabolism
Bustany et al. 1985	6	Unknown	3 medicated, 3 drug naive	^{11}C$_L$-methionine	Frontal hypometabolism of protein synthesis
Jernigan et al. 1985	6	Auditory vigilance task, eyes closed	Off > 2 weeks	^{18}F-deoxyglucose	No difference in frontal ratio analysis
Wolkin et al. 1985	10	Resting, eyes open, ears plugged	Off > 2 weeks	^{18}F-deoxyglucose	Reduced absolute frontal metabolism but no difference in frontal ratio analysis before treatment; reduced relative prefrontal glucose metabolism after treatment
Kling et al. 1986	6	Eyes open, lying in scanner	All medicated	^{18}F-deoxyglucose	No difference in frontal ratio analysis

Volkow et al. 1986	4	Resting	3 never medicated, 1 treated for 3 months 12 months prior to study	^{11}C-2-deoxyglucose	No difference in frontal ratio analysis
Cohen et al. 1987	16	Auditory vigilance task	Off > 13 days	^{18}F-deoxyglucose	Reduced absolute prefrontal glucose metabolism
Early et al. 1987	10	Resting, eyes closed	Drug naive	^{15}O	No difference in prefrontal or CBF ratio analysis
Gur et al. 1987	12	Eyes and ears open	7 off > 6 months or drug naive, 5 had 7–10 days drug washout	^{18}F-deoxyglucose	No difference in absolute or relative frontal glucose metabolism
Kishimoto et al. 1987	20	Resting, eyes closed	17 on haloperidol	^{11}C-glucose	Hypofrontal pattern in 6 patients, hypoparietal pattern in 8 patients, normal pattern in 6 patients
Volkow et al. 1987	18	1) Resting; 2) eye tracking	All medicated	^{11}C-deoxyglucose	Reduced absolute and relative prefrontal glucose metabolism under both conditions

(continued)

Table 4–11. Controlled PET studies evaluating frontal metabolism in schizophrenia (continued)

Study	Schizophrenic sample size	Test conditions	Medication status	Metabolic tracer	Results
Wiesel et al. 1987	20	Resting, eyes covered	Off > 3 weeks; off depot > 6 months	^{11}C-glucose	No difference in frontal ratio analysis
Szechtman et al. 1988	15	Resting, eyes closed	All medicated	^{18}F-deoxyglucose	Increased relative frontal glucose metabolism
Wolkin et al. 1988	13	Eyes open, ears plugged	Off > 2 weeks	^{18}F-deoxyglucose	Reduced absolute and relative frontal glucose metabolism
Cleghorn et al. 1989	8	Resting, eyes closed	Drug naive	^{18}F-deoxyglucose	Increased relative frontal glucose metabolism
Buchsbaum 1990	13	Continuous performance task	All off > 31 days (mean = 30 weeks)	^{18}F-deoxyglucose	Reduced absolute and relative frontal glucose metabolism

The studies summarized in Tables 4–10 and 4–11 illustrate a steady progression in sophistication. Early studies tended to examine chronic patients, to evaluate the "resting state," and to explore relatively small samples. Sometimes patients were studied while neuroleptic free, but not always. In later studies, investigators recognized that study of the resting state has specific limitations; it is difficult to say what the human brain actually does when it is "resting." Consequently, strategies have been employed to produce consistencies across individuals, such as the delivery of a painful stimulus. More importantly, however, a paradigm involving the use of at least two back-to-back conditions has also been developed. In this strategy, an experimental task is identified that has been selected because it is assumed to stimulate the prefrontal cortex. Examples include the Wisconsin Card Sorting Test, the Continuous Performance Test, the Porteus Mazes, and the Tower of London. A baseline or control task is selected to control for as many components of the activation task as possible. When the baseline condition is subtracted from the activation condition, selective activation (or failure to activate) in the prefrontal cortex can be identified.

Unfortunately, very few studies have evaluated hypofrontality in relation to clinical phenomenology. Most studies have simply identified patients with schizophrenia as defined using DSM-III or DSM-III-R. Thus, most studies are essentially showing a relationship between hypofrontality and the diagnosis of schizophrenia, without an attempt to determine whether there is any relationship between hypofrontality and prominent negative symptoms. A relationship was noted, however, in the early studies by Franzen and Ingvar (1975a, 1975b).

In our research program at the University of Iowa, we recently completed a systematic study that explored the issue of hypofrontality in schizophrenia using a design that built on the work of previous investigators (Andreasen et al. 1993). In this study, we identified two different patient groups: 1) drug-naive, first-admission patients and 2) chronically ill schizophrenic patients who had been withdrawn from medication for a 3-week period. Because at least one PET study has reported that drug-naive patients may in fact be hyperfrontal, a concern has been raised that hypofrontality could simply be an epiphenomenon, caused by long-term treatment with neuroleptic drugs. The specific design that we employed allowed us to explore the effects of chronicity on hypofrontality relatively independently of the effects of medication.

The first group evaluated in our study consisted of 13 "neuroleptic-naive" schizophrenic patients; that is, they had never been treated with any type of neuroleptic drug. This naive status was assessed through a careful clinical history obtained from the family, the patient, and any prior medical records that were available. The second sample consisted of 27 nonnaive schizophrenic patients who had been relatively chronically ill. They were admitted to the University of Iowa Mental Health Clinical Research Center and taken off their medication for a 3-week period prior to scanning. These two groups did not differ significantly from one another in any variables of interest, such as educational achievement, age, or gender composition. The two groups of patients were compared with a group of 15 normal control subjects recruited from the community. The control subjects were selected to match the schizophrenic patients as closely as possible for age, gender, and educational status of parents.

The patients were systematically evaluated at the Mental Health Clinical Research Center using a variety of standard rating instruments, including the CASH, the SANS, the SAPS, the Global Assessment Scale (Endicott et al. 1976), the Hamilton Rating Scale for Depression (Hamilton 1960), the Abnormal Involuntary Movement Scale (Department of Health, Education and Welfare 1974), and the Simpson Angus Scale (Simpson and Angus 1970). Measurements of the severity of positive and negative symptoms were obtained on the day that imaging studies were done, to achieve the potentially most valid correlations between severity of symptoms and measures of brain physiology. All patients were medication free at the time these assessments were obtained, thus ensuring that any negative symptoms observed were not secondary to the effects of medication.

All patients were scanned using the ^{133}Xe method to measure regional cerebral blood flow. Scans were done on a Tomomatic 64 (Medimatic) and measurements of regional cerebral blood flow were generated based on the method of Kanno and Lassen (1979). Cerebral perfusion studies were conducted back-to-back for each subject over a 25-minute time period (each scan takes approximately 4 minutes, with a resting period of 15 minutes between studies). The initial study was done under a baseline condition; the second study was done while the subjects were given an experimental cognitive challenge, the Tower of London.

We selected the Tower of London as a cognitive challenge because it seemed to have a variety of desirable characteristics for physiological imaging. The time window of ^{133}Xe studies is 4 minutes. An ideal task is one that remains relatively the same throughout the imaging period. The Tower of London is a sequential planning task that challenges the subject to figure out how to move a series of balls lined up on a stick to a final predetermined goal position, using three adjacent sticks. The task has variable difficulty, with easy levels requiring only two moves and more difficult levels requiring five or six moves. Nevertheless, the task is relatively simple, and it was selected because it was one that most schizophrenic patients were relatively able to perform. The Tower of London assesses the subject's ability to formulate a plan and complete it, a cognitive function that is considered to be mediated through the prefrontal cortex. Its relevance to the prefrontal cortex has been partially validated through the work of Shallice (1982).

Because the performance of the task involves manipulating colored shapes observed on a video monitor, we developed a baseline condition that would recruit many of the same brain regions that are involved in the experimental task. During the baseline condition, subjects were asked to watch undulating colored shapes on a video monitor. We hypothesized that this baseline condition would activate visual and right parietal function, regions that would also be recruited during the performance of the Tower of London. Thus this baseline condition permitted us to use image math techniques; by subtracting the baseline condition from the cognitive activation condition, we could identify which regions were selectively activated in normal individuals. Thereafter, we could determine whether these regions performed in the same way or differently in schizophrenic patients.

Tables 4–12 and 4–13 show image subtraction data for five specific regions of interest that were measured in this study. As these tables indicate, the three groups differed significantly in perfusion to only two regions: left mesial frontal and right parietal. The normal control subjects showed an increase in left mesial frontal flow in relation to the rest of the brain when given the cognitive challenge, whereas the two patient groups showed a decrease. Dunnett's post hoc test found that the drug-naive patients were significantly different from the control subjects. The other area showing a significant difference was the right parietal cortex. The control subjects showed a substantial increase in flow to this region in relation to the rest of the brain, whereas the two patient groups showed little difference. In this case, the Dunnett's post hoc test indicated that both groups of patients differed significantly from the control subjects.

These data indicate that hypofrontality is present in first-episode patients who have never received neuroleptic treatment. They allow us to infer that hypofrontality is therefore not secondary to the effects of either medication or chronicity. We were also interested in determining

Table 4–12. Left-hemisphere localization scores for control subjects, drug-naive patients, and drug-nonnaive patients

	Control subjects		Drug-naive patients		Drug-nonnaive patients	
	Mean	SD	Mean	SD	Mean	SD
Mesial frontal activation	9.02	8.72	5.48	13.41	5.08	10.51
Hemisphere activation	7.32	8.59	9.44	9.96	6.63	8.47
Localization	1.70	5.15	-3.96	5.62	-1.55	6.28
Lateral frontal activation	5.49	11.29	8.49	12.00	7.20	9.92
Hemisphere activation	7.71	8.24	9.07	10.18	6.39	8.46
Localization	-2.23	4.85	-0.59	5.62	0.82	4.81
Temporal activation	4.60	8.21	8.85	10.59	4.57	8.52
Hemisphere activation	8.11	8.74	9.05	10.47	6.86	8.83
Localization	-3.51	4.90	-0.21	6.03	-2.29	5.93
Parietal activation	9.28	7.08	11.62	8.96	6.81	7.56
Hemisphere activation	6.97	9.10	9.05	10.47	6.36	9.24
Localization	2.31	4.52	3.39	4.78	0.45	6.13
Occipital activation	6.11	10.35	9.94	10.71	6.85	10.92
Hemisphere activation	7.74	8.29	8.87	10.57	6.40	8.25
Localization	-1.63	4.69	1.08	7.79	0.44	5.16

Table 4–13. Right-hemisphere localization scores for control subjects, drug-naive patients, and drug-nonnaive patients

	Control subjects		Drug-naive patients		Drug-nonnaive patients	
	Mean	SD	Mean	SD	Mean	SD
Mesial frontal activation	7.99	8.66	10.63	11.77	6.03	10.21
Hemisphere activation	7.86	9.17	10.34	9.49	7.97	8.35
Localization	0.13	5.20	0.29	7.09	-1.94	6.68
Lateral frontal activation	6.56	9.86	8.45	9.03	7.45	9.57
Hemisphere activation	8.01	8.94	10.57	9.60	7.79	8.35
Localization	-1.45	3.62	-2.12	3.05	-0.34	5.55
Temporal activation	5.20	12.32	8.08	9.73	5.35	8.28
Hemisphere activation	8.42	8.63	10.84	9.88	8.26	8.82
Localization	-3.22	7.21	-2.77	6.84	-2.91	7.07
Parietal activation	10.36	8.65	10.70	8.49	7.85	8.14
Hemisphere activation	7.12	9.29	10.27	9.89	7.73	8.51
Localization	3.24	4.19	0.43	2.81	0.12	3.20
Occipital activation	8.57	10.48	12.04	12.87	10.60	11.75
Hemisphere activation	7.75	8.84	10.09	9.10	7.29	8.15
Localization	0.81	4.27	1.95	5.84	3.32	7.82

whether any relationship could be observed between negative symptoms and hypofrontality. Thus we divided the entire group of patients into two subgroups based on their ratings of negative symptoms on the day that the scan was done. Patients who had a negative symptom rating of 4 or greater for two symptoms (using global ratings for alogia, affective blunting, anhedonia, and avolition) were classified as having prominent negative symptoms. The remainder of the patients were placed in the other group. For these analyses, all patients were pooled together, because sample size was not sufficient to produce adequate power if the two groups of patients were analyzed separately. The results of these analyses are shown in Table 4–14. As the table indicates, patients with prominent negative symptoms do not show an increase in perfusion to the left mesial prefrontal cortex while performing the Tower of London; on the other hand, the normal controls and the "low negative" patients do show prefrontal increases in perfusion.

This study permitted us to assess hypofrontality in schizophrenia in relation to a variety of variables, such as effects of long-term treatment, chronicity of illness, and presenting phenomenology. We were able to demonstrate that hypofrontality is not secondary to either treatment or chronicity, but that it is related to severity of negative symptoms, since decreased activation occurred only in the "high negative" group.

References

American Psychiatric Association: Diagnostic and Statistical Manual of Mental Disorders, 3rd Edition. Washington, DC, American Psychiatric Association, 1980

American Psychiatric Association: Diagnostic and Statistical Manual of Mental Disorders, 3rd Edition, Revised. Washington, DC, American Psychiatric Association, 1987

Andreasen NC: Negative symptoms in schizophrenia: definition and reliability. Arch Gen Psychiatry 39:784–788, 1982

Andreasen NC: The Scale for the Assessment of Negative Symptoms (SANS). Iowa City, The University of Iowa, 1983

Andreasen NC: The Scale for the Assessment of Positive Symptoms (SAPS). Iowa City, The University of Iowa, 1984

Andreasen NC: Comprehensive Assessment of Symptoms and History (CASH). Iowa City, The University of Iowa, 1985a

Andreasen NC: Positive vs. negative schizophrenia: a critical evaluation. Schizophr Bull 11:380–389, 1985b

Table 4–14. Relationship between negative symptoms and cerebral blood flow in frontal cortex

| | Left hemisphere | | | | | | Right hemisphere | | | | | |
| | Lateral | | | Mesial | | | Lateral | | | Mesial | | |
Group[a]	Base	Activation	> t	Base	Activation	> t	Base	Activation	> t	Base	Activation	> t
Control (slice 4)												
Mean	75.80	82.93	*	83.27	95.00	***	75.60	83.13	**	87.67	95.87	**
SD	11.23	13.16		15.38	15.23		11.73	12.43		16.87	15.68	
Low symptomatology												
Mean	75.81	84.50	***	92.38	98.50	NS	76.19	87.00	***	90.06	99.44	***
SD	11.12	12.95		16.01	14.53		13.46	14.24		15.33	17.23	
High symptomatology												
Mean	75.85	82.95	*	89.05	94.10	NS	75.50	81.95	*	87.60	94.75	*
SD	14.11	15.08		18.83	17.90		12.36	15.75		18.45	18.68	
Control (weighted average from all slices)												
Mean	77.57	83.06	*	81.44	90.46	***	78.20	84.76	*	83.97	91.96	**
SD	12.00	11.58		14.59	12.89		11.95	11.85		15.41	14.0	

(continued)

Table 4–14. Relationship between negative symptoms and cerebral blood flow in frontal cortex *(continued)*

| | Left hemisphere | | | | | | Right hemisphere | | | | | |
| | Lateral | | | Mesial | | | Lateral | | | Mesial | | |
Group[a]	Base	Activation	> t	Base	Activation	> t	Base	Activation	> t	Base	Activation	> t
Low symptomatology												
Mean	77.84	86.54	***	89.03	95.60	**	79.74	87.73	***	87.43	96.72	***
SD	12.11	11.39		13.63	12.40		14.12	13.73		13.95	15.29	
High symptomatology												
Mean	77.51	84.35	*	87.52	91.67	NS	78.26	85.93	***	86.70	93.11	*
SD	14.17	13.69		17.59	15.70		13.36	14.02		17.47	16.97	

Note. Patients were classified as having high negative symptoms if they scored 4 or higher on at least two of the global ratings for affective blunting, alogia, anhedonia, or avolition on the Scale for the Assessment of Negative Symptoms. All other patients were classified as having low negative symptomatology. NS = not significant.

[a]Control $n = 15$; low symptomatology $n = 16$; high symptomatology $n = 20$.

* $P < .005$, one-tailed; ** $P < .01$, one-tailed; *** $P < .001$, one-tailed.

Andreasen NC: The Scale for the Assessment of Negative Symptoms (SANS): conceptual and theoretical foundations. Br J Psychiatry 155 (suppl 7):49–52, 1989

Andreasen NC: Positive and negative symptoms: historical and conceptual aspects, in Modern Problems of Pharmacopsychiatry: Positive and Negative Symptoms and Syndromes. Edited by Andreasen NC. Basel, Karger, 1990, pp 1–42

Andreasen NC, Flaum M: Schizophrenia: the characteristic symptoms. Schizophr Bull 17:27–49, 1990

Andreasen NC, Grove WM: Evaluation of positive and negative symptoms in schizophrenia. Psychiatrie et Psychobiologie 2:108–121, 1986

Andreasen NC, Olson S: Negative versus positive schizophrenia: definition and validation. Arch Gen Psychiatry 39:789–794, 1982

Andreasen NC, Flaum M, Arndt S: The Comprehensive Assessment of Symptoms and History (CASH): an instrument for assessing psychopathology and diagnosis. Arch Gen Psychiatry 49:615–623, 1992

Andreasen NC, Rezai K, Alliger R, et al: Hypofrontality in neuroleptic-naive and chronic schizophrenic patients: assessment with xenon-133 single photon emission computed tomography and the Tower of London. Arch Gen Psychiatry 49:943–958, 1993

Ariel RN, Golden CJ, Berg RA, et al: Regional cerebral blood flow in schizophrenics. Arch Gen Psych 40:258–263, 1983

Arndt S, Alliger RJ, Andreasen NC: The distinction of positive and negative symptoms: the failure of a two-dimensional model. Br J Psychiatry 158:317–322, 1991

Bajc M, Medved V, Basic M, et al: Cerebral perfusion inhomogeneities in schizophrenia demonstrated with single photon emission computed tomography and Tc99m-hexamethylpropyleneamineoxim. Acta Psychiatr Scand 80:427–433, 1989

Berman KF, Zec RF, Weinberger DR: Physiologic dysfunction of dorsolateral prefrontal cortex in schizophrenia, II: role of neuroleptic treatment, attention, and mental effort. Arch Gen Psychiatry 43:126–135, 1986

Berman KF, Illowsky BP, Weinberger DR: Physiological dysfunction of dorsolateral prefrontal cortex in schizophrenia, IV: further evidence for regional and behavioral specificity. Arch Gen Psychiatry 45:616–622, 1988

Bilder RM, Mukherjee S, Rieder RO, et al: Symptomatic and neuropsychological components of defect states. Schizophr Bull 11:409–419, 1985

Buchsbaum MS: The frontal lobes, basal ganglia, and temporal lobes as sites for schizophrenia. Schizophr Bull 16:379–389, 1990

Buchsbaum MS, Ingvar DH, Kessler R, et al: Cerebral glucography with positron tomography. Arch Gen Psychiatry 39:251–259, 1982

Buchsbaum MS, DeLisi LE, Holcomb HH, et al: Anteroposterior gradients in cerebral glucose use in schizophrenia and affective disorders. Arch Gen Psychiatry 41:1159–1166, 1984

Bustany P, Henry JF, Rotrou JD, et al: Correlations between clinical state and positron emission tomography measurement of local brain protein synthesis in Alzheimer's dementia, Parkinson's disease, schizophrenia, and gliomas, in The Metabolism of the Human Brain Studied With Positron Emission Tomography. Edited by Greitz T, Ingvar DH, Widen L. New York, Raven, 1985, pp 241–251

Chabrol H, Guell A, Bes A, et al: Cerebral blood flow in schizophrenic adolescents. Am J Psychiatry 143:130, 1986

Cleghorn JM, Garnett ES, Nahmias C, et al: Increased frontal and reduced parietal glucose metabolism in acute untreated schizophrenia. Psychiatry Res 28:119–133, 1989

Cohen RM, Gross M, Nordahl TE, et al: Dysfunction in a prefrontal substrate of sustained attention in schizophrenia. Life Sci 40:2031–2039, 1987

Cohen RM, Semple WE, Gross M, et al: Evidence for common alterations in cerebral glucose metabolism in major affective disorders and schizophrenia. Neuropsychopharmacology 2:241–254, 1989

Cummings JL, Mendez MF: Secondary mania with focal cerebrovascular lesions. Am J Psychiatry 141:1084–1087, 1984

Department of Health, Education and Welfare: Abnormal Involuntary Movement Scale. Washington, DC, U.S. Department of Health, Education and Welfare, Alcohol, Drug Abuse and Mental Health Administration, 1974

Devous MD Sr, Raese JD, Herman JH, et al: Regional cerebral blood flow in schizophrenic patients at rest and during Wisconsin card sort tasks. J Cereb Blood Flow Metab 5 (suppl 1):S201–S202, 1985

Dousse M, Mamo H, Ponsin JC, et al: Cerebral blood flow in schizophrenia. Exp Neurol 199:98–111, 1988

Early TS, Reiman EM, Raichle ME, et al: Left globus pallidus abnormality in never-medicated patients with schizophrenia. Proc Natl Acad Sci U S A 84:561–563, 1987

Endicott J, Spitzer RL, Fleiss JL, et al: The Global Assessment Scale: a procedure for measuring overall severity of psychiatric disturbances. Arch Gen Psychiatry 33:766–771, 1976

Erbas B, Kumbasar H, Erbengi G, et al: Tc-99m HMPAO/SPECT determination of regional cerebral blood flow changes in schizophrenics. Clin Nucl Med 12:904–907, 1990

Farkas T, Wolf AP, Jaeger J, et al: Regional brain glucose metabolism in chronic schizophrenia: a positron emission transaxial tomographic study. Arch Gen Psychiatry 41:293–300, 1984

Franzen G, Ingvar DH: Abnormal distribution of cerebral activity in chronic schizophrenia. J Psychiatr Res 12:199–214, 1975a

Franzen G, Ingvar DH: Absence of activation in frontal structures during psychological testing of chronic schizophrenics. J Neurol Neurosurg Psychiatry 38:1027–1032, 1975b

Freud S: Project for a scientific psychology (1895), in The Standard Edition of the Complete Psychological Works of Sigmund Freud. Translated and edited by Strachey J. London, Hogarth Press, 1966, pp 283–398

Fuster JM: The Prefrontal Cortex: Anatomy, Physiology, and Neuropsychology of the Frontal Lobe, 2nd edition. New York, Raven, 1989

Geraud G, Arne-Bes MC, Guell A, et al: Reversibility of hemodynamic hypofrontality in schizophrenia. J Cereb Blood Flow Metab 7(1):9–12, 1987

Goldman-Rakic P: The frontal lobes: unchartered provinces of the brain (special issue). Trends Neurosci 7(11), 1984

Guenther W, Moser E, Mueller-Spahn F, et al: Pathological cerebral blood flow during motor function in schizophrenic and endogenous depressed patients. Biol Psychiatry 21:889–899, 1986

Gur RE, Skolnick BE, Gur RC, et al: Brain function in psychiatric disorders, I: regional cerebral blood flow in medicated schizophrenics. Arch Gen Psychiatry 40:1250–1254, 1983

Gur RE, Gur RC, Skolnick BE, et al: Brain function in psychiatric disorders, III: regional cerebral blood flow in unmedicated schizophrenics. Arch Gen Psychiatry 42:329–334, 1985

Gur RE, Resnick SM, Alavi A, et al: Regional brain function in schizophrenia, I: a positron emission tomography study. Arch Gen Psychiatry 44:119–125, 1987

Hamilton M: A rating scale for depression. J Neurol Neurosurg Psychiatry 23:56–62, 1960

Heaton R: Wisconsin Card Sorting Test. Odessa, TX, Psychological Assessment Resources, 1985

Humbert M, Salvador L, Segul J, et al: Estudio interfiabilidad version espanola evaluacion de sintomas positivos y negativos. Rev Departmento Psiquiatria Facultad de Medicina, University of Barcelona 13:28–36, 1986

Ingvar DH, Franzen G: Abnormalities of cerebral blood flow distribution in patients with chronic schizophrenia. Acta Psychiatr Scand 50:425–462, 1974

Jernigan TL, Sargent T, Pfefferbaum A, et al: 18-Fluorodeoxyglucose PET in schizophrenia. Psychiatry Res 16:317–329, 1985

Kanno I, Lassen NA: Two methods for calculating cerebral blood flow from emission computed tomography in inert gas concentrations. J Comput Assist Tomogr 3:71–76, 1979

Kety SS, Woodford RB, Harmel MH, et al: Cerebral blood flow and metabolism in schizophrenia: the effects of barbiturate semi-narcosis, insulin coma and electroshock. Am J Psychiatry 104:765–770, 1948

Kishimoto H, Kuwahara H, Ohno S, et al: Three subtypes of chronic schizophrenia identified using 11C-glucose positron emission tomography. Psychiatry Res 21:285–292, 1987

Kling AS, Metter EJ, Riege WH, et al: Comparison of PET measurement of local brain glucose metabolism and CAT measurement of brain atrophy in chronic schizophrenia and depression. Am J Psychiatry 143:175–180, 1986

Kraepelin E: Dementia Praecox and Paraphrenia. Translated by Barclay RM, Robertson GM. Edinburgh, E&S Livingstone, 1919

Kurachi M, Kobayashi K, Matsubara R, et al: Regional cerebral blood flow in schizophrenic disorders. Eur Neurol 24:176–181, 1985

Liddle PF: The symptoms of chronic schizophrenia: a re-examination of the positive-negative dichotomy. Br J Psychiatry 151:145–151, 1987

Mathew RJ, Meyer JS, Francis DJ, et al: Regional cerebral blood flow in schizophrenia: a preliminary report. Am J Psychiatry 138:112–113, 1981

Mathew RJ, Duncan GC, Weinman ML, et al: Regional cerebral blood flow in schizophrenia. Arch Gen Psychiatry 39:1121–1124, 1982

Mathew RJ, Wilson WH, Tant SR, et al: Abnormal resting regional cerebral blood flow patterns and their correlates in schizophrenia. Arch Gen Psychiatry 45:542–549, 1988

McGorry PD, Copolov DL, Singh BS: Royal Park Multidiagnostic Instrument for Psychosis, I: rationale and review. Schizophr Bull 16:501–515, 1990a

McGorry PD, Singh BS, Copolov DL, et al: Royal Park Multidiagnostic Instrument for Psychosis, II: development, reliability, and validity. Schizophr Bull 16:501–515, 1990b

Moscarelli M, Maffei C, Cesana BM: An international perspective on assessment of negative and positive symptoms in schizophrenia. Am J Psychiatry 144:1595–1598, 1987

Ohta T, Okazaki Y, Anzai N: Reliability of the Japanese version of the Scale for the Assessment of Negative Symptoms (SANS). Japanese Journal of Psychiatry 13:999–1010, 1984

Paulman RG, Devous MD, Gregory RR, et al: Hypofrontality and cognitive impairment in schizophrenia: dynamic single-photon tomography and neuropsychological assessment of schizophrenic brain function. Biol Psychiatry 27:377–399, 1990

Sagawa K, Kawakatsu S, Shibuya I, et al: Correlation of regional cerebral blood flow with performance on neuropsychological tests in schizophrenic patients. Schizophr Res 3:241–246, 1990

Shallice T: Specific impairments of planning. Philos Trans R Soc London 298:199–209, 1982

Sheppard G, Gruzelier J, Manchanda R, et al: 15-O Positron emission tomographic scanning in predominantly never-treated acute schizophrenic patients. Lancet 24/31:1448–1452, 1983

Simpson GM, Angus JWS: A rating scale for extrapyramidal side effects. Acta Psychiatr Scand 1 (suppl):212, 1970

Szechtman H, Nahmias C, Garnett S, et al: Effect of neuroleptics on altered cerebral glucose metabolism in schizophrenia. Arch Gen Psychiatry 45:523–532, 1988

Volkow ND, Brodie JD, Wolf AP, et al: Brain metabolism in patients with schizophrenia before and during neuroleptic administration. J Neurol Neurosurg Psychiatry 49:1199–1202, 1986

Volkow ND, Wolf AP, Van Gelder P, et al: Phenomenological correlates of metabolic activity in 18 patients with chronic schizophrenia. Am J Psychiatry 144:151–158, 1987

Warkentin S, Nilsson A, Karlson S, et al: Regional cerebral blood flow in schizophrenia and cycloid psychosis. J Cereb Blood Flow Metab 5 (suppl 1):S185–S186, 1985

Warkentin S, Nilsson A, Risberg J, et al: Regional cerebral blood flow in schizophrenia: repeated studies during a psychotic episode. Psychiatry Res: Neuroimaging 35:27–38, 1990

Weinberger DR, Berman KF, Zec RF: Physiological dysfunction of dorsolateral prefrontal cortex in schizophrenia, I: regional cerebral blood flow (rCBF) evidence. Arch Gen Psychiatry 43:114–124, 1986

Weinberger DR, Berman KF, Illowsky BP: Physiological dysfunction of dorsolateral prefrontal cortex in schizophrenia, III: a new cohort and evidence for a monoaminergic mechanism. Arch Gen Psychiatry 45:609–615, 1988

Wiesel FA, Wik G, Sjogren I, et al: Altered relationships between metabolic rates of glucose in brain regions of schizophrenic patients. Acta Psychiatr Scand 76:642–647, 1987

Wittgenstein L: The Blue Book. Oxford, Basil Blackwell, 1958

Wolkin A, Jaeger J, Brodie JD, et al: Persistence of cerebral metabolic abnormalities in chronic schizophrenia as determined by positron emission tomography. Am J Psychiatry 142:564–571, 1985

Wolkin A, Angrist B, Wolf A, et al: Low frontal glucose utilization in chronic schizophrenia: a replication study. Am J Psychiatry 145:251–253, 1988

Wood FB, Flowers DL: Hypofrontal vs. hypo-Sylvian blood flow in schizophrenia. Schizophr Bull 16:413–424, 1990

Chapter 5

Brain Function in Schizophrenia

Application of Neurobehavioral Studies

Ruben C. Gur, Ph.D.
Andrew J. Saykin, Psy.D.
Raquel E. Gur, M.D., Ph.D.

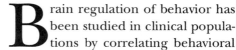

B rain regulation of behavior has been studied in clinical populations by correlating behavioral deficits with clinical signs, postmortem findings, and, more recently, neuroimaging data. The surge of interest in the neurosciences and the emergence of neuroimaging techniques have provided an unprecedented opportunity to examine the neurobiology of schizophrenia. This has resulted in increased application of neurobehavioral data in the search for brain regions that may be dysfunctional in schizophrenia.

Linking regional brain function with behavioral dimensions has traditionally been accomplished by application of behavioral measures to

This investigation was supported by NIMH Grants MH43880, MH42191, and MH00586. We thank Drs. Arthur Benton, Edith Kaplan, and Harvey Levin for their collaboration on the behavioral imaging project and D. Brian Kester, M.A., and Margaret Taleff, M.S., for their assistance.

patients with brain disease and, more recently, neurophysiologic "activation" procedures. These combined strategies can help describe how a behavioral measure is "mapped" in the brain. They all serve the aim of understanding how behavior is regulated by brain mechanisms and networks.

Nature and Measured Dimensions of Neuropsychological Batteries

Neuropsychological batteries include a broad range of behavioral measures, such as abstraction, reasoning, language, memory, spatial skills, and sensorimotor integration. The batteries were designed for and have been applied primarily in the diagnosis and characterization of the behavioral consequences of brain lesions in neurologic and neurosurgical populations. In these patients brain dysfunction can be inferred from the pattern of deficit.

The application of neuropsychological tests has usually included administration of a standard set or "battery" of tests. There have been two major trends regarding selection of measures in neuropsychological research with clinical batteries: the "fixed" and the "flexible" battery approaches (Incagnoli et al. 1986). Fixed batteries include comprehensive sets of tests such as the Halstead-Reitan (Reitan and Wolfson 1985) and the Luria-Nebraska neuropsychological batteries (Golden et al. 1980). In contrast, the flexible approach (Benton and Hamsher 1976; Benton et al. 1983; Goodglass 1986; Milberg et al. 1986) usually involves a core battery, with additional sampling of selected functional domains used to test specific hypotheses (Goodglass 1986; Luria 1966; Milberg et al. 1986). Either approach permits comparison of performance of patients with schizophrenia with performance of patients with other brain disorders.

Structural brain lesions typically affect a functional system (Luria 1966) or network (Mesulam 1981). In schizophrenia, and other brain disorders, a number of dimensions of brain function have been examined. Anterior lesions, affecting the frontal brain system, can disrupt most higher-level cognitive operations by causing a disorganization of goal-directed behavior, particularly related to attentional processing and conceptual flexibility (E. Goldberg and Bilder 1987; T. E. Goldberg et al. 1987; Perecman 1987; Stuss et al. 1982). Often identified as "executive" deficits, frontal lobe impairment can affect multiple processes. Psychometrically, these deficits appear on the Wisconsin Card Sorting Test

(Grant and Berg 1948; Heaton 1981), Trail-Making B (Reitan and Wolfson 1985), and measures of verbal or figural fluency.

In contrast, temporal lobe lesions, particularly of the medial temporal lobe region (which includes the hippocampus and amygdala), are associated with deficits in memory and learning of new information (Squire and Butters 1984). In humans, this has been studied most closely in the context of surgical treatment of medically refractory seizure disorders (Milner 1975). During the acute postoperative phase after left medial temporal lobe resections, patients frequently show deficits in verbal memory for prose passages and in learning lists of information. The California Verbal Learning Test (Delis et al. 1983) and the Wechsler Memory Scale (Russell 1975; Wechsler 1945) are sensitive to these acute changes (Milner 1975; Saykin et al. 1991). As expected from theories on hemispheric specialization of function, deficits have been observed in nonverbal memory for designs, faces, and musical sequences after right medial temporal lobe resections.

Subcortical systems have been implicated in a number of diseases (Ricklin and Levita 1969), and subcortical dementia has received increasing attention. Neuroimaging studies in schizophrenia have examined the basal ganglia because of the dopamine-rich connections to the frontal lobes and the pattern of activity, which covaries with the patient's pharmacologic status. Perceptual-motor integration, fine motor skills, spatial ability, and procedural memory are putative neurobehavioral functions of the basal ganglia. There are presently no neuropsychological tests that are pathognomonic for basal ganglia involvement. In spite of this absence of specificity, many tests tapping the abilities just described appear sensitive to basal ganglia dysfunction.

Application of Neuropsychological Batteries to Schizophrenia

Standard neuropsychological tests have been widely applied in studies of patients with schizophrenia. The results have generally demonstrated diffuse impairment as indicated by cognitive, perceptual, and attentional deficits on a range of instruments (Goldstein 1986; Heaton et al. 1978; Levin et al. 1989; Malec 1978; Saykin et al. 1991; Seidman 1983). Across studies, patients with schizophrenia have performed poorly on complex cognitive and perceptual tests that pose high demands on information-processing systems involved in maintenance of attention and exercise of rapid psychomotor speed (Goldstein 1986).

There have been several regional hypotheses in the neuropsychology of schizophrenia examining the dimensions described in the preceding section: anterior/posterior, left/right, and cortical/subcortical. Involvement of anterior brain systems, particularly the frontal lobes, has been suggested by deficits in higher-level abstraction and mental flexibility on tests such as the Wisconsin Card Sorting Test and the Halstead Category Test (Berman et al. 1986; Flor-Henry and Yeudall 1979; Flor-Henry et al. 1983; T. E. Goldberg et al. 1987; Weinberger et al. 1986, 1988). Involvement of the left hemisphere has been implicated by deficits in verbal cognitive functions, such as low Verbal Intelligence Quotient (VIQ) relative to Performance Intelligence Quotient (PIQ) and impairment on language tests (Andreasen 1979a, 1979b; Andreasen and Grove 1979; Flor-Henry and Yeudall 1979; Newlin et al. 1981; Silverberg-Shalev et al. 1981). Subcortical and cortical dysfunction has been implicated by studies of attention and information processing (Mirsky 1977, 1986). The extensive interconnectivity between the frontal lobes and diencephalic limbic and reticular structures makes subcortical systems potential sites for disruption of attentional processes via impaired selective gating of information (Skinner and Lindsley 1973). Mesulam (1981, 1985) proposed a neural network for attention, which involves parietal, temporal, and frontal cortex as well as the cingulate gyrus and subcortical "limbic" regions. Attentional deficits, also noted in genetic studies of children of patients with schizophrenia, may provide a biological marker (Erlenmeyer-Kimling et al. 1989; Nuechterlein and Dawson 1984).

Methodological Issues in Data Interpretation

Methodological problems in early psychometric studies were encountered (Heaton and Crowley 1981). Some are unique to schizophrenia, but others are common to clinical populations. The conceptual basis for applying neurobehavioral methods was often superficial, attempting to separate patients with "functional" schizophrenia from those with organic brain dysfunction. The general finding has been that the level of performance of schizophrenic patients falls between that of patients with known structural brain lesions and that of control samples.

However, the interpretation of the obtained deficits is complicated by a number of psychometric problems, particularly the formation and analysis of quantitative profiles and the mapping of these profiles onto regional brain systems. As is evident, both frontal lobe functions, including abstraction and attention, and temporal lobe functions, including learning and memory, are impaired in schizophrenia. This, however, is a part of the general impairment, which spares only a few simple functions. The question becomes, first, how to test which function is differentially impaired (Chapman and Chapman 1989) and, second, what are the implications of such differential impairment to hypotheses on regional brain dysfunction.

This is a complicated undertaking for several reasons. To establish that function A is differentially impaired, it is necessary to administer not only a test for function A, but tests for all other candidate functions as well as measures of general ability. This raises the logistical demand to balance the need for comprehensive evaluation against what is practical for a patient. Furthermore, as Chapman and Chapman (1989) emphasized, the various measures must have comparable reliability and task difficulty for healthy subjects. Otherwise we can be misled to infer that a patient is impaired in test A and not test B, upon finding a significant effect for A and not for B, when the only reason for this is that test A is more reliable and hence more sensitive to effects of pathology.

Another dilemma is how to deal with education. It could be argued whether education correlates with brain anatomic or metabolic measures, but without doubt education is an important factor in evaluating neuropsychological test performance. When studying the effects of a focal brain disease acquired late in life, such as stroke, it makes sense to balance patients and control subjects for educational attainment. On the other hand, schizophrenia is a developmental disease affecting individuals while they are in the midst of achieving their educational goals, and it directly interferes with the attainment of these goals. Because reduced educational attainment is a part of the syndrome, it would be a "matching fallacy" (Meehl 1970) to equate patients and control subjects for education. A more appropriate variable to use for balancing the samples is parental education. However, the effects of education do need to be examined, and perhaps in some cases partialed out, to interpret differences between patients and control subjects.

Finally, it is important to bear in mind that the disease itself affects behavior on many levels other than the cognitive performance assessed by neuropsychological testing. The patient's motivation, cooperation, and psychotic symptoms and their treatment should all be considered.

We have attempted to address some of these methodological issues through two avenues. First, we have examined the functional characterization of deficits in an unmedicated sample (Saykin et al. 1991), as described in the next section of this chapter. Second, we have begun to apply regional analyses of the neuropsychological data using an algorithm for topographic display and analysis of the test scores (R. C. Gur et al. 1988a, 1988b, 1990; Trivedi and Gur 1987, 1989).

Functional Analysis of Deficits

We have applied a battery that measures a range of behavioral functions and implicated brain regions. From this battery it is possible to test specific hypotheses, such as frontal relative to temporal lobe impairment in schizophrenia, by contrasting performance of the same patients on the functions associated with these brain regions. Specifically, the frontal lobe hypothesis predicts that patients will show selective impairment on the Wisconsin Card Sorting Test, whereas the temporal lobe hypothesis predicts selective impairment on the memory and learning tests.

In a sample of 36 patients and 36 healthy control subjects (Saykin et al. 1991), we found that patients were impaired in both abstraction (Wisconsin Card Sorting Test) and memory tests. However, the impairment in memory and learning was significantly greater than the impairment on the Wisconsin Card Sorting Test. This effect, which supports a selective temporal lobe deficit in schizophrenia, remained when variables that might affect performance were considered in the statistical analysis. It existed for both men and women, across the age range (which was 18–45 years), for all educational levels, and for both highly cooperative and less cooperative patients.

It is still questionable whether we can conclude, on the basis of this effect alone, that the temporal lobes are differentially affected in schizophrenia whereas the frontal lobes are not. How do abstraction and memory compare with other functions? Conceivably both could be superior or inferior to the general level of performance. We compared each to the other functions using a profile analysis and found that abstraction was significantly better in patients relative to their average neuropsychological performance, whereas memory and learning were significantly worse than all other functions (Saykin et al. 1991).

Even this strong form of support for the temporal lobe hypothesis relative to the frontal lobe hypothesis does not settle the issue of identifying specific regional brain dysfunction. The memory deficit could be ubiquitous and robust and may indeed point to temporal lobe dysfunction, and yet a constellation of other deficits can suggest other brain regions that may be implicated. There is a need for a systematic evaluation of the combined set of neuropsychological data in relation to current theory of brain behavior regulation. This will permit the identification of impaired neural networks.

The nature of the brain disease we expect to find in schizophrenia is not a focal lesion with circumscribed boundaries and effects, but more likely involves neurotransmitter systems with distributed physiologic effects. Given that, it would be a mistake to find an area of greatest abnormality and declare it as the "site of schizophrenia." Rather, we will have to continue the investigative effort, searching systematically for networks. This requires the joining of neuropsychological test scores with hypotheses linking them to the integrity of all regions of interest. We have developed an algorithm, "behavioral imaging," which attempts to accomplish this by providing standard regional interpretation of neuropsychological measures.

Behavioral Imaging

The process of testing neurobehavioral theories is assisted by a quantification of theories concerning regional brain involvement in the regulation of behavior. The algorithm that we have proposed applies such a quantification to standard neuropsychological test scores (Trivedi and Gur 1987, 1989). The algorithm yields values for specific brain regions, which reflect the prediction that the region is dysfunctional given a pattern of neuropsychological scores. The regional values can also be presented topographically to facilitate comprehension of the spatial distribution of implicated brain areas.

The algorithm applies weights for each test score × region, reflecting the rated sensitivity of the score for a lesion in this area. The weights are multiplied by the scores obtained, and the intensity of a pixel is a function of the summed product normalized for the sum of weights assigned for a given region (R. C. Gur et al. 1988a). The weights were supplied by expert neuropsychologists and showed inter-expert agreement and intra-expert reliability (R. C. Gur et al. 1990).

Initial testing of the algorithm in clinical cases and populations was encouraging (R. C. Gur et al. 1988a, 1988b). There was consistency between the "behavioral images" and the location of lesions in patients with unilateral cerebral infarcts. The topographic displays showed correspondence with clinical, computed tomography (CT), and metabolic data and were congruent with the clinical interpretation of the neuropsychological assessment. Patients with focal ischemic lesions have been a major source of information on the validity of neurobehavioral theories. This is because of the circumscribed nature of many infarcts, and the tendency of such lesions to occur in adult, neurally mature brains. The potential of the algorithm was also evaluated in a sample of patients with hemiparkinsonism (Blonder et al. 1989; R. C. Gur et al. 1988b). The hypothesis of greater neurobehavioral deficits associated with the hemisphere ipsilateral to the side of striatal deficiency was supported. We are currently evaluating the algorithm in other clinical populations with focal and diffuse brain disorders.

Conclusions

In our search for brain mechanisms that may explain the pathophysiology of schizophrenia, neurobehavioral studies can play an important role. The neuropsychology of "mental" disorders is a relatively new field, and there is an opportunity to properly orient its course. There should be a generally accepted "core" procedure for obtaining neuropsychological data. The individuals administering this battery must be supervised by qualified neuropsychologists and trained in the specialized application of neuropsychological tests to psychiatric populations. The main purpose of neuropsychological testing is not for differential diagnosis of schizophrenia. Its purpose is to assess and characterize the pattern of behavioral impairment and preserved abilities. It quantifies the pervasiveness of impairment and can help determine the degree of brain dysfunction. This is important for assessing progression, medication effects, and rehabilitation.

In addition to the application of test batteries, such as those described in this chapter, there is potential for advancing the field using combined behavioral and physiologic studies. The activation paradigm appears to be a more appropriate model for schizophrenia. It provides physiologic data when individuals are engaged in neurobehavioral tasks that are known to activate specific brain regions in healthy subjects. This paradigm has been applied to the study of schizophrenia to examine the laterality hypothesis (R. E. Gur et al. 1983, 1985) and the frontal lobe dysfunction hypothesis (Berman et al. 1986; Weinberger et al. 1986). This is, however, only the beginning of what could become a productive line of research that will generate more refined understanding of the neurobehavioral substrates of schizophrenia.

References

Andreasen NC: Thought, language and communication disorders, I: clinical assessment, definition of terms and evaluation of their reliability. Arch Gen Psychiatry 36:1315–1321, 1979a

Andreasen NC: Thought, language and communication disorders, II: diagnostic significance. Arch Gen Psychiatry 36:1325–1330,1979b

Andreasen NC, Grove W: The relationship between schizophrenic language, manic language and aphasia, in Hemispheric Asymmetries in Function in Psychopathology. Edited by Gruzelier J, Flor-Henry P. Amsterdam, Elsevier-North Holland, 1979, pp 373–390

Benton AL, Hamsher K: Multilingual Aphasia Examination. Iowa City, University of Iowa, 1976

Benton AL, Hamsher K, Varney N, et al: Contributions to Neuropsychological Assessment: A Clinical Manual. New York, Oxford University Press, 1983

Berman KF, Zec RF, Weinberger DR: Physiologic dysfunction of dorsolateral prefrontal cortex in schizophrenia, II: role of neuroleptic treatment, attention, and mental effort. Arch Gen Psychiatry 43:126–135, 1986

Blonder LX, Gur RE, Gur RC, et al: Neuropsychological functioning in hemiparkinsonism. Brain Cogn 9:177–190, 1989.

Chapman LJ, Chapman JP: Strategies for resolving the heterogeneity of schizophrenics and their relatives using cognitive measures. J Abnorm Psychol 98:357–366, 1989

Delis DC, Kramer JH, Kaplan EF, et al: California Verbal Learning Test, Manual. New York, The Psychological Corporation (Harcourt Brace Jovanovich), 1983

Erlenmeyer-Kimling L, Golden RR, Cornblatt BA: A taxometric analysis of cognitive and neuromotor variables in children at risk for schizophrenia. J Abnorm Psychol 98:203–208, 1989

Flor-Henry P, Yeudall LT: Neuropsychological investigations of schizophrenia and manic-depressive psychoses, in Hemispheric Asymmetries of Function in Psychopathology. Edited by Gruzelier J, Flor-Henry P. Amsterdam, Elsevier-North Holland, 1979, pp 341–362

Flor-Henry P, Fromm-Auch D, Schopflocher D: Neuropsychological dimensions in psychopathology, in Laterality and Psychopathology. Edited by Flor-Henry P, Gruzelier J. Amsterdam, Elsevier Bio-Medical, 1983, pp 59–82

Goldberg E, Bilder R Jr: The frontal lobes and hierarchical organization of cognitive control, in The Frontal Lobes Revisited. Edited by Perecman E. New York, IRBN Press, 1987, pp 159–187

Goldberg TE, Weinberger DR, Berman KF, et al: Further evidence for dementia of the prefrontal type in schizophrenia? a controlled study of teaching the Wisconsin Card Sorting Test. Arch Gen Psychiatry 44:1008–1014, 1987

Golden CJ, Hammeke TA, Purisch AD: Manual, Luria-Nebraska Neuropsychological Battery. Los Angeles, CA, Western Psychological Services, 1980

Goldstein G: The neuropsychology of schizophrenia, in Neuropsychological Assessment of Neuropsychiatric Disorders. Edited by Grant I, Adams KM. New York, Oxford University Press, 1986, pp 147–171

Goodglass H: The flexible battery in neuropsychological assessment, in Clinical Application of Neuropsychological Batteries. Edited by Incagnoli T, Goldstein G, Golden CJ. New York, Plenum, 1986, pp 121–134

Grant DA, Berg EA: A behavioral analysis of degree of reinforcement and ease of shifting to new responses in a Weigl-type card sorting problem. J Exp Psychol 38:404–411, 1948

Gur RC, Trivedi SS, Saykin AJ, et al: "Behavioral imaging"—a procedure for analysis and display of neuropsychological test scores, I: construction of algorithm and initial clinical application. Neuropsychiatry, Neuropsychology and Behavioral Neurology 1:53–60, 1988a

Gur RC, Saykin AJ, Blonder LX, et al: "Behavioral imaging", II: application of the quantitative algorithm to hypothesis testing in a population of hemiparkinsonian patients. Neuropsychiatry, Neuropsychology and Behavioral Neurology 1:87–96, 1988b

Gur RC, Saykin AJ, Benton A, et al: "Behavioral imaging", III: inter-rater agreement and reliability of weightings. Neuropsychiatry, Neuropsychology and Behavioral Neurology 3:113–124, 1990

Gur RE, Skolnick BE, Gur RC, et al: Brain function in psychiatric disorders, I: regional cerebral blood flow in medicated schizophrenics. Arch Gen Psychiatry 40:1250–1254, 1983

Gur RE, Gur RC, Skolnick BE, et al: Brain function in psychiatric disorders, III: regional cerebral blood flow in unmedicated schizophrenics. Arch Gen Psychiatry 42:329–334, 1985

Heaton RK: Wisconsin Card Sorting Test, Manual. Odessa, TX, Psychological Assessment Resources, 1981

Heaton RK, Crowley TJ: Effects of psychiatric disorders and their somatic treatments on neuropsychological test results, in Handbook of Clinical Neuropsychology. Edited by Filskov SB, Boll TJ. New York, Wiley-Interscience, 1981

Heaton RK, Baade LE, Johnson KL: Neuropsychological test results associated with psychiatric disorders in adults. Psychol Bull 85:141–162, 1978

Incagnoli T, Goldstein G, Golden CJ (eds): Clinical Application of Neuropsychological Batteries. New York, Plenum, 1986

Levin S, Yurgelun-Todd D, Craft S: Contributions of clinical neuropsychology to the study of schizophrenia. J Abnorm Psychol 98:341–356, 1989

Luria AR: Higher Cortical Functions in Man. New York, Basic Books, 1966

Malec J: Neuropsychological assessment of schizophrenia versus brain damage: a review. J Nerv Ment Dis 166:507–516, 1978

Meehl PE: Nuisance variable and the ex post facto design, in Minnesota Studies in the Philosophy of Science. Edited by Radner M, Winokur S. Minneapolis, University of Minnesota Press, 1970, pp 373–402

Mesulam M-M: A cortical network for directed attention and unilateral neglect. Ann Neurol 10:309–325, 1981

Mesulam M-M (ed): Principles of Behavioral Neurology. Philadelphia, PA, FA Davis, 1985

Milberg WP, Hebben N, Kaplan E: The Boston process approach to neuropsychological assessment, in Neuropsychological Assessment of Neuropsychiatric Disorders. Edited by Grant I, Adams KM. New York, Oxford University Press, 1986, pp 65–86

Milner B: Psychological aspects of focal epilepsy and its neurosurgical management. Advanced Neurology, Vol 8. New York, Raven, 1975, pp 299–321

Mirsky AF: Behavioral and electrographic measures of attention in children at risk for schizophrenia. J Abnorm Psychol 86:27–33, 1977

Mirsky AF: From Worcester to Haifa: fifty years of attention research in neuropsychiatry. Paper presented at the annual meeting of the American Psychological Association, Washington, DC, 1986

Newlin DB, Carpenter B, Golden CJ: Hemispheric asymmetries in schizophrenia. Biol Psychiatry 16:561–582, 1981

Nuechterlein KH, Dawson ME: Information processing and attention in the developmental course of schizophrenic disorders. Schizophr Bull 10:160–203, 1984

Perecman E (ed): The Frontal Lobes Revisited. New York, IRBN Press, 1987

Reitan RM, Wolfson D: The Halstead-Reitan Neuropsychological Test Battery: Theory and Clinical Interpretation. Tucson, AZ, Neuropsychology Press, 1985

Ricklin ML, Levita E: Subcortical Correlates of Human Behavior. Baltimore, MD, Williams & Wilkins, 1969

Russell EW: A multiple scoring method for assessment of complex memory functions. J Consult Clin Psychol 43:800–809, 1975

Saykin AJ, Gur RC, Gur RE, et al: Neuropsychological function in schizophrenia: selective impairment in memory and learning. Arch Gen Psychiatry 4:618–624, 1991

Seidman L: Schizophrenia and brain dysfunction: an integration of recent neurodiagnostic findings. Psychol Bull 94:195–238, 1983

Silverberg-Shalev R, Gordon HW, Bentin S, et al: Selective language deterioration in chronic schizophrenia. J Neurol Neurosurg Psychiatry 44:547–551, 1981

Skinner JE, Lindsley DB: The nonspecific mediothalamic-frontocortical system: its influence on electrocortical activity and behavior, in Psychophysiology of the Frontal Lobes. Edited by Pribram KH, Luria AR. New York, Academic Press, 1973

Squire LR, Butters N: Neuropsychology of Memory. New York, Guilford, 1984

Stuss DT, Kaplan EF, Benson DF, et al: Evidence for the involvement of orbitofrontal cortex in memory functions: an interference effect. Journal of Comparative and Physiological Psychology 96:913–925, 1982

Trivedi SS, Gur RC: Computer graphics for neuropsychological data. Proceedings of the National Computer Graphics Association 3:22–32, 1987

Trivedi SS, Gur RC: Topographic mapping of cerebral blood flow and behavior. Comput Biol Med 19:219–229, 1989

Wechsler DA: A standardized memory scale for clinical use. J Psychol 19:87–95, 1945

Weinberger DR, Berman KF, Zec RF: Physiologic dysfunction of dorsolateral prefrontal cortex in schizophrenia, I: regional cerebral blood flow evidence. Arch Gen Psychiatry 43:114–124, 1986

Weinberger DR, Berman KF, Illowsky BP: Physiological dysfunction of dorsolateral prefrontal cortex in schizophrenia, III: a new cohort and evidence for a monoaminergic mechanism. Arch Gen Psychiatry 45:609–615, 1988

Chapter 6

Phenomenology, Environmental Risk, and Genetics
Twin Studies of Schizophrenia

Adrianne M. Reveley, M.D.

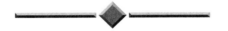

Twins, particularly identical twins, have always provoked interest. For the past hundred years science has employed twins as a useful natural experiment to try to disentangle the effects of genes and environment, but for centuries past they have been celebrated in literature and the theater. Shakespeare often used them as a dramatic device—perhaps not surprisingly as he was himself the father of twins. *The Comedy of Errors* includes two pairs, and in *Twelfth Night* Sebastian and Viola are twins: "one face, one voice, one habit and two persons" (Shakespeare apparently did not know that identical twins should always be the same sex).

Three centuries after Shakespeare, Sir Francis Galton (1883) pioneered the use of twins in scientific research, quoting the Shakespearean phrase "nature vs nurture" (from *The Tempest*) in his intuitive suggestion, made without knowledge of the biology of zygosity differences, that identical and fraternal twins might be compared to look at "the relative effects of nature and nurture on disposition and intellectual ability." Galton was interested in the tendency of "genius" (by which he meant giftedness in one capacity or another) to appear regularly through the generations in certain distinguished families like his own.

Phenomenology and Genetics

The Classic Twin Studies

Thirty years after Kraepelin developed the first modern definition of schizophrenia, his former trainee Luxenberger (1928), at the Munich School of Psychiatric Genetics, undertook the first twin study of schizophrenia. This was actually the first twin study of any psychiatric disorder. The aim of this and the later classic twin studies was to establish the genetic contribution to schizophrenia and to confirm the distinction between schizophrenia and manic-depressive disorder.

Luxenberger recognized the value of complete ascertainment to avoid an overrepresentation of identical and/or concordant pairs, and he identified all 16,382 patients in the Munich Psychiatric Clinic and the populations of 12 Bavarian mental hospitals on a given day. He then systematically surveyed the birth records of these patients for twin birth. He was able to show quite convincingly that twinship was no more frequent among psychotic patients than among the general population. In his study he deliberately restricted himself to strict Kraepelinian dementia praecox in both twin and co-twin, which might explain the lack of concordant dizygotic pairs in his series, and he jettisoned all pairs from the analysis where only one was available or zygosity was uncertain.

There followed a series of twin studies of schizophrenia (Table 6–1), which systematically surveyed chronic inpatients. In the first phase of twin research up to the time of the Second World War, the genetic contribution to schizophrenia and its distinction from manic-depressive disorder seemed established. In the largest series, Kallmann (1946) found no case

Table 6–1.   Twin studies of schizophrenia: systematic surveys of chronic psychiatric inpatients

Study	MZ	% Concordance	DZ	% Concordance
Luxenberger 1928	19	58	13	0
Essen-Möller 1941	11	64	27	15
Kallmann 1946	174	69	296	10
Slater 1953	37	65	58	14

Note. MZ = monozygotic. DZ = dizygotic.
Source. Data from Gottesman and Shields 1982.

where a schizophrenic proband had an identical manic-depressive co-twin, and through later years this finding has remained broadly true.

Meanwhile, the phase of early twin research in schizophrenia ended with the critical work of Rosenthal (1959). He predicted that studies taken from a general population base, rather than surveys of inpatients, would find lower concordance rates for schizophrenia for a number of reasons, such as overreporting of concordant cases, and overweighting of samples with severe cases, and he was, of course, proved right (Table 6–2). Tables 6–1 and 6–2 are based on those constructed by Gottesman and Shields (1982), who have contributed so much to our understanding of the strengths and limitations of the various twin studies of schizophrenia.

Up to this point in schizophrenia research the phenomenological picture was murky, with reliance on a consensus of experts, or merely established practice, to make a diagnosis. Some twin studies were spoiled by a failure to present the full material, and few allowed an investigation of the finer nuances of phenomenology. Gottesman and Shields (1972), working in the 1960s on the Maudsley Twin Register, sought to incorporate all known methodological refinements and provided summaries that have been extensively used as source material for further studies (Table 6–3).

The Maudsley Twins

The Bethlehem Royal Hospital, now joint with the Maudsley Hospital, goes back about 900 years, with systematic patient records collected from the 17th century. The Maudsley Twin Register was set up by Eliot Slater in 1948 (Slater 1953) by the simple process of incorporating a

Table 6–2. Twin studies of schizophrenia: population-based studies using probandwise concordance

Study	MZ	% Concordance	DZ	% Concordance
Kringlen 1967	55	45	90	15
Tienari 1971	17	35	20	13
Pollin et al. 1969	95	43	125	9
Fischer 1973	21	56	41	27

Note. MZ = monozygotic. DZ = dizygotic.
Source. Data from Gottesman and Shields 1982.

question about twinship on the routine demographic data sheet filled out for every patient. Thus all patients attending any psychiatric facility of the joint hospitals are checked for twinship, and the records of those responding positively are sent on to the Genetics Section where twin and co-twin are followed up. The information available in the records is extensive, as the traditions of the Maudsley ensure careful longitudinal and phenomenological scrutiny. Of all Maudsley patients, 1.96% were born one of twins (Chitkara et al. 1988), and the register now stands at over 2,000 pairs with psychiatric disorder in one or both.

No twin study has so far been completed that set out to use modern diagnostic criteria, but the summaries prepared by Gottesman and Shields on the Maudsley twins are suitable for the criteria to be applied post hoc. Studies using this series are summarized in Table 6–3. Robins and Guze (1970) were the first to point out that since the best etiological contributors to schizophrenia are genes, the diagnostic scheme that shows that the highest heritability is likely to have the greatest validity. In 1984 we used the Gottesman and Shields summaries in this way (McGuffin et al. 1984). The strategy was surprisingly successful and reinforces the validity of modern criteria as well as the soundness of the twin method. However, without the certainty of a biological indicator of schizophrenia, diagnostic criteria tend to reflect the thinking in psychiatry at the time that they are developed. Modern criteria are more strin-

Table 6–3.   Studies of twins consecutively registered at the Maudsley Hospital, 1948–1963

Diagnostic system (study)	MZ	% Concordance	DZ	% Concordance
Expert's consensus (Gottesman and Shields 1972)	22	58	33	12
"Severe" schizophrenia (Gottesman and Shields 1972)	11	55	24	8
Research Diagnostic Criteria (McGuffin et al. 1984)	22	45	23	9
DSM-III (Farmer et al. 1987)	21	48	21	10

Note.   MZ = monozygotic. DZ = dizygotic.
Source.   Data from Gottesman and Shields 1972.

gent than the psychiatric thinking of the 1960s. Of the original 69 cases of schizophrenia in the Gottesman and Shields series, Research Diagnostic Criteria (RDC) reduce them to 49 cases, with a similar reduction for DSM-III (American Psychiatric Association 1980; Farmer et al. 1987).

In 1982 we described a case of identical triplets, of whom two apparently had schizophrenia (diagnosed on the basis of continuous auditory hallucinations and poor social functioning) and one had manic-depressive disorder (McGuffin et al. 1982). These triplets have been followed up since that time. One of those originally diagnosed schizophrenic gradually improved until he was asymptomatic on neuroleptics. He married a fellow patient and asked for medication to be stopped because of sexual dysfunction. Six weeks after stopping depot neuroleptics, he was brought to the hospital with a clear-cut episode of mania with flight of ideas, grandiosity, and lack of sleep. His symptoms have responded well to lithium. Although changes from schizophrenia to manic-depressive disorder are more uncommon than the other way around, they are not unknown, and they emphasize our continuing uncertainty about the relationship between these disorders (e.g., Crow 1990).

Environmental Risk and Twins

One of the great attractions of studying twins is that discordant monozygotic twins provide an apparently perfect control for the effect of genes. The co-twin control method introduced by Gesell and Thompson (1929) is simple in principle—if both twins have the same genes but differ with respect to a characteristic, then environment must be responsible for the difference between them. Recently it has become clear that this is a generalization, as identical twins can be genetically different in some circumstances (Burn 1988), but the method still has merit. For co-twin control investigations, unlike phenomenological studies, there is no virtue in a consecutive series. Much may be learned by comparing discordant twin and co-twin, even more by comparing them with concordant pairs.

Birth Weight

The co-twin control method was first applied to birth weight in schizophrenia in the late 1960s (Table 6–4). The results are inconsistent, but the consensus of the studies suggests that the lighter twin is the most at risk. We have extended the method to show that discordant pairs may differ from concordant pairs by having greater intrapair birth weight differences, whether or not the ill twin was the lighter, suggesting that more complex interuterine or developmental factors may be implicated (Lewis et al. 1987).

Cerebral Ventricular Size

The co-twin control method can be uniquely useful in investigating biological markers. The platelet monoamine oxidase (MAO) story is well known following Murphy and Wyatt's original observation in 1972. Theirs was the first co-twin control study of a biological marker in schizophrenia. It showed that the well co-twins also had low MAO compared with control subjects, though not as low as the schizophrenic subjects, suggesting that the medication was not entirely responsible for low platelet MAO in schizophrenia. We followed and extended their method and obtained almost exactly the same results (M. A. Reveley et al. 1983).

The same group of twins that we used in our 1983 study were the subjects for the first co-twin control study of brain structure in schizophrenia (A. M. Reveley et al. 1982). Using computed tomography (CT), we compared ventricular size in members of discordant pairs, and we also compared the affected and unaffected twins with monozygotic control subjects. The schizophrenic subjects had consistently larger cerebral ventricles than their identical co-twins, but both had larger lateral ventricles than the control twins. In our investigations of control twins, we found ventricular size to be under a high degree of genetic control, with similar

Table 6–4.   Birth weights in discordant psychotic monozygotic twins

Study	Ill twin lighter (pairs)	Ill twin heavier (pairs)	Equal weights (pairs)
Tienari 1963	8	6	0
Kringlen 1967	9	12	4
Mosher et al. 1971	12	3	0
Gottesman and Shields 1972	5	0	2
Lewis et al. 1987	7	3	3
Totals	41	24	9

heritabilities derived from monozygotic and dizygotic groups of around 0.80 (A. M. Reveley et al. 1984a). The family study by DeLisi et al. (1986) supports this result. These findings suggest the following conclusions:

1. Anatomical changes in the brain are associated with schizophrenia.
2. The pathogenesis of such changes cannot be entirely genetic.
3. Since the unaffected co-twins of the schizophrenic subjects differed significantly from the control series, some genetic diathesis for these changes may provide a substrate that interacts with environmental insult.

These conclusions have recently been supported to some extent (Table 6–5) by data using magnetic resonance imaging (MRI) in 15 pairs of discordant schizophrenic twins, from the National Institute of Mental Health brain imaging group (Suddath et al. 1990). Again, the schizophrenic twin from monozygotic discordant pairs was significantly more likely to have larger cerebral ventricles. MRI allows more detailed investigation of brain structure than CT, and the investigators were able to look at the hippocampus and temporal lobe. They found that the affected twins had smaller hippocampi. Unfortunately, although Suddath et al. examined intrapair differences in seven sets of normal control twins, they did not compare the control twins with the schizophrenic subjects and their discordant co-twins, nor did they attempt intrapair correlations in their control series. Thus it is impossible to say if the unaffected twins differed from the control series of twins or if hippocampal or temporal lobe size appeared to be under genetic control among control twins. This omission might not seem important or significant were it not for our finding that birth injury and low birth weight were significantly associated with ventricular size in control subjects, but not in schizophrenic twins (A. M. Reveley et al. 1984a, 1984b), suggesting that ventricular enlargement in schizophrenia is of complex etiology and may even be partly genetic.

We went on to show (Tables 6–6 and 6–7) in a series of twin and nontwin schizophrenic and control subjects (A. M. Reveley and Reveley 1987) that increased ventricular size was more significantly associated with twinning than it was with schizophrenia. This suggests that increased cerebral ventricular size is a peripheral indicator of the cerebral pathology involved in schizophrenia. It also raises questions as to the suitability of twins for schizophrenia research.

Table 6–5. Brain imaging studies in discordant schizophrenic twins

Study	Method	Population	Findings
A. M. Reveley et al. 1982	Computed tomography	10 discordant MZ, with MZ, DZ, and schizophrenic nontwin controls	• VBR highly heritable in normal twins • VBR significantly larger in schizophrenic twins than in MZ co-twins • Lack of usual density ratio in schizophrenic twins • VBR larger in healthy twins than in singletons
Suddath et al. 1990	Magnetic resonance imaging	15 discordant MZ twins	• Left temporal gray matter reduced in schizophrenic twins vs. co-twins • Lateral ventricles larger in schizophrenic twins vs. co-twins

Note. MZ = monozygotic. DZ = dizygotic. VBR = ventricular brain ratio.

Twin-Specific Abnormalities: Limitations of the Twin Method

It is tempting to go back to the old literature, which cautioned against the use of twins because they might have an excess of schizophrenia on the basis of cerebral injury or developmental problems, or because the twinning process itself disturbs laterality and so renders the twins more liable to laterality-related disorders. Rosanoff et al. (1934–1935) were the first to raise cautions about the use of twins, followed more recently by Campion and Tucker (1973) and Boklage (1977).

It is certainly true that twins are more at risk than singletons in a number of ways and for specific conditions, some of which seem to be related to obstetric complications, others to disturbed laterality (Table 6–8). Even the causes of monozygotic twinning, apart from the very rare dominant form, suggest disadvantage, and such twins may not even be identical genetically (Burn 1988). Is schizophrenia one of the conditions found more often among twins?

Twin Susceptibility to Schizophrenia

Boklage (1977) suggested, in a reanalysis of handedness in the Gottesman and Shields series, that disturbed laterality, presenting as "non-righthandedness," might contribute to discordance in schizophrenia.

Table 6–6. Ventricular brain ratio (VBR) in control subjects

Group	N	Sex ratio	Age	VBR
Monozygotic twins	14	1.33	32 ± 7.0	4.8 ± 2.7
Dizygotic twins	17	1.43	34 ± 5.6	6.2 ± 2.8
Singletons	44	1.32	33 ± 6.5	3.9 ± 2.5

Note. $P > .01$, twin versus singleton.

Table 6–7. Ventricular brain ratio (VBR) in schizophrenic subjects

Group	N	Sex ratio	Age	IQ (MillHill)	VBR
Monozygotic twins	25	1.27	39 ± 12	34 ± 35	7.2 ± 4.7
Singletons	25	0.8	40 ± 12	28 ± 29	5.2 ± 2.8

Note. $P > .05$, twin versus singleton.

There are conflicting reports on handedness in twins, but handedness is a very poor indicator of laterality. Other, better indicators, such as dermatoglyphic patterns and hair whorl direction, suggest that twins are likely to suffer altered laterality. They also have an increase in congenital malformations, particularly cardiac malformations, which depend on abnormal laterality during embryogenesis for their development (Burn 1988). There have been two other studies of handedness in discordant schizophrenic twins (Lewis et al. 1989; Luchins et al. 1980), neither of which showed a significant association between handedness and discordance.

The possibility remains that twins might be more susceptible to schizophrenia on the basis of obstetric complications. There is no doubt that twins are more susceptible to obstetric complications and to premature birth than are singletons (reviewed in Chitkara et al. 1988), but how significant is this in relation to schizophrenia? Recent evidence seems to favor the idea that obstetric complications may themselves relate to preexisting abnormality in the fetus, which renders the fetus less able to participate in the birth process (Goodman 1988).

An easy way to resolve the difficulty is to see if twins are overrepresented among samples of schizophrenic patients. I have already referred to Luxenberger (1928), who found that 1.7% of the psychotic individuals whom he investigated were twins, compared with 1.8% of the general Munich population. Table 6–9 shows more recent studies, including one from our group. None show a significant excess of twins except for one category—that of twins whose co-twins died in the perinatal period, which we have called "co-twin dead."

Table 6–8. Conditions for which twins are more at risk than singletons

- Lower birth weight: monozygotic < dizygotic (Corney et al. 1972)
- Maternal preeclampsia (MacGillivray et al. 1982)
- Premature birth: monozygotic > dizygotic, males > females (Corney et al. 1983)
- Perinatal morbidity and mortality (for a review, see Chitkara et al. 1988)
- Survivor damage after twin death (e.g., microcephaly) (D'Alton et al. 1984)
- Neural tube defects (× 1.8) (Windham and Bjerkedal 1984)
- Cardiac malformation (× 1.7) (Burn and Corney 1984)
- Disturbed lateralization (e.g., Burn 1988)

In our study (Chitkara et al. 1988), we started with a base population of 25,663 Maudsley patients and categorized them by ICD-9 casenote diagnosis using a hierarchical system over time, so that the category "schizophrenia" really means "ever achieved schizophrenia," and so on. There was a nonsignificant excess of twins among the schizophrenia, personality disorder, and substance abuse groups. Turning to the much smaller "co-twin dead" group and looking at their distribution among the twin sample, we found that they were significantly overrepresented in the same three groups. For unknown reasons, co-twin dead twins are more likely to be male, but the effect of gender is not sufficient to explain the phenomenon. The peculiar excess of schizophrenia in twins whose co-twin died at birth remains unexplained, although the most simplistic explanation would be susceptibility on the basis of some factor that caused the death of one twin and schizophrenia in the other.

Other evidence suggests that twin susceptibility to schizophrenia on the basis of some adverse environmental event is unlikely, based on the almost equal likelihood that the offspring of the well twin of a discordant pair will be affected with schizophrenia as the offspring of the ill twin. Gottesman and Bertelsen (1989) studied the offspring of the Fischer series of twins and found that the morbid risk in offspring of ill twins was 16.8% and the morbid risk in offspring of well co-twins was 17.4%, compared with rates of 17.4% and 2.1% in the offspring of discordant fraternal twins.

Table 6–9. Studies of the association of schizophrenia with twinning

Study	Sample	Findings
Pollin et al. 1969	VA twin sample	0.96% schizophrenic twins among MZ twins, 1.22% schizophrenic twins among DZ twins (males only, comparable to the general population)
Gottesman and Shields 1972	Maudsley twin series 1949–1951	2.18% of all hospital patients are twins
Chitkara et al. 1988	Maudsley twin series 1967–1978	1.96% of 20,895 hospital are twins; nonsignificant excess of twins among 1,500 schizophrenic patients (2.4%); significant excess of "co-twin dead at birth" among schizophrenic twins

Note. VA = Veterans Administration. MZ = monozygotic. DZ = dizygotic.

Conclusion

Twins have made and will continue to make a unique contribution to our understanding of schizophrenia. They offer one of the few validators of clinical "caseness" and phenomenology. The co-twin control studies extend the twin method, offering a unique way to understand biological markers. Although twins are at risk for congenital abnormalities associated with lateralization failure, they do not appear to be at risk for schizophrenia. However, further study of the elusive relationship between twinning, brain organization, and schizophrenia may offer the greatest reward in our attempt to understand the development of psychosis.

References

American Psychiatric Association: Diagnostic and Statistical Manual of Mental Disorders, 3rd Edition. Washington, DC, American Psychiatric Association, 1980

Boklage CE: Schizophrenia, brain asymmetry development, and twinning: cellular relationships with etiological and possibly prognostic implications. Biol Psychiatry 12:19–35, 1977

Burn J: Monozygotic twins, in Contemporary Obstetrics and Gynecology. Edited by Chamberlain G. Stoneham, MA, Butterworth-Heinemann, 1988

Burn J, Corney G: Congenital heart defects and twinning. Acta Genet Med Gemellol (Roma) 33:61–69, 1984

Campion E, Tucker G: A note on twin studies, schizophrenia and neurological impairment. Arch Gen Psychiatry 29:460–464, 1973

Chitkara B, Reveley AM, Macdonald AM: Twin birth and adult psychiatric disorder: an examination of the case records of the Maudsley Hospital. Br J Psychiatry 152:391–398, 1988

Corney G, Robson EB, Strong SJ: The effect of zygosity on the birth weight of twins. Ann Hum Genet 36:45–59, 1972

Corney G, MacGillivray I, Campbell DM, et al: Congenital abnormalities in twins in Aberdeen and North East Scotland. Acta Genet Med Gemellol (Roma) 32:31–35, 1983

Crow TJ: The continuum of psychosis and its genetic origins. Br J Psychiatry 156:788–797, 1990

D'Alton ME, Newton ER, Cetrulo CL: Interuterine fetal demise in multiple gestation. Acta Genet Med Gemellol (Roma) 33:43–49, 1984

DeLisi LE, Goldin CR, Hamovit JR, et al: A family study of the association of increased ventricular size with schizophrenia. Arch Gen Psychiatry 43:148–153, 1986

Essen-Möller E: Psychiatrische Untersuchungen an einer Serie von Zwillingen. Acta Psychiatr et Neurol Suppl 23:1–200, 1941

Farmer AE, McGuffin P, Gottesman II: Twin concordance for DSM-III schizophrenia: scrutinizing the validity of the definition. Arch Gen Psychiatry 44:634–641, 1987

Fischer M: Genetic and environmental factors in schizophrenia: a study of schizophrenic twins and their families. Acta Psychiatr Scand Suppl 238:9–142, 1973

Galton F: Inquiries Into Human Faculty. London, Macmillan, 1883

Gesell A, Thompson H: Learning and growth in identical infant twins: an experimental study by the method of co-twin control. Genetic Psychology Monographs 6:5–124, 1929

Goodman R: Are complications of pregnancy and birth causes of schizophrenia? Dev Med Child Neurol 30:391–406, 1988

Gottesman II, Bertelson A: Confirming unexpressed genotypes for schizophrenia. Arch Gen Psychiatry 46:867–872, 1989

Gottesman II, Shields J: Schizophrenia and Genetics: A Twin Study Vantage Point. London, Academic Press, 1972

Gottesman II, Shields J: Schizophrenia: The Epigenetic Puzzle. Cambridge, Cambridge University Press, 1982

Kallmann FJ: The genetic theory of schizophrenia: an analysis of 691 schizophrenic twin index families. Am J Psychiatry 103:309–322, 1946

Kringlen E: Heredity and Environment in the Functional Psychoses. London, Heinemann, 1967

Lewis SW, Chitkara B, Reveley AM, et al: Family history and birthweight in monozygotic twins concordant and discordant for psychosis. Acta Genet Med Gemellol (Roma) 36:267–272, 1987

Lewis SW, Chitkara B, Reveley AM: Hand preference in psychotic twins. Biol Psychiatry 25:215–221, 1989

Luchins DJ, Pollin W, Wyatt RJ: Laterality in monozygotic twins: an alternative hypothesis. Biol Psychiatry 15:87–93, 1980

Luxenberger H: Vorlaufiger Bericht uber Psychiatrische Serien Untersuchungen an Zwillingen: Zeitschrift fur die Gesamte Neurologie und Psychiatrie 116:297–326, 1928

MacGillivray I, Campbell DM, Samphier M, et al: Preterm deliveries in twin pregnancies in Aberdeen. Acta Genet Med Gemellol (Roma) 31:207–211, 1982

McGuffin P, Reveley AM, Holland A: Identical triplets—non-identical psychosis. Br J Psychiatry 140:1–6, 1982

McGuffin P, Farmer AE, Gottesman II, et al: Twin concordance for operationally defined schizophrenia. Arch Gen Psychiatry 41:541–545, 1984

Murphy DL, Wyatt RJ: Reduced platelet monoamine oxidase activity in blood platelets from schizophrenic patients. Nature 238:225–226, 1972

Pollin W, Allen MG, Hoffer A, et al: Psychopathology in 15,909 pairs of veteran twins. Am J Psychiatry 7:597–609, 1969

Reveley AM, Reveley MA: The relationship of twinning to the familial-sporadic distinction in schizophrenia. J Psychiatr Res 21:515–520, 1987

Reveley AM, Reveley MA, Clifford CA, et al: Cerebral ventricular size in twins discordant for schizophrenia. Lancet 1:540–541, 1982

Reveley AM, Reveley MA, Murrays RM: Cerebral ventricular enlargement in non-genetic schizophrenia: a controlled twin study. Br J Psychiatry 144:89–93, 1984a

Reveley AM, Reveley MA, Chitkara B, et al: The genetic basis of cerebral ventricular volume. Psychiatry Res 13:261–266, 1984b

Reveley MA, Reveley AM, Clifford CA, et al: The genetics of platelet MAO activity in schizophrenic and normal twins. Br J Psychiatry 142:560–565, 1983

Robins E, Guze SB: Establishment of diagnostic validity in psychiatric illness: its application to schizophrenia. Am J Psychiatry 126:983–987, 1970

Rosanoff AJ, Handy LM, Plesset IR, et al: The etiology of so-called schizophrenic psychoses with special reference to their occurrence in twins. Am J Psychiatry 91:247–286, 1934–1935

Rosenthal D: Some factors associated with concordance and discordance with respect to schizophrenia in monozygotic twins. J Nerv Ment Dis 129:1–10, 1959

Slater E: Psychotic and Neurotic Illnesses in Twins. Medical Research Council Special Report Series No 278. London, Her Majesty's Stationery Office, 1953

Suddath RL, Christison GW, Torrey EF, et al: Anatomical abnormalities in the brains of monozygotic twins discordant for schizophrenia. N Engl J Med 322:789–794, 1990

Tienari P: Schizophrenia and monozygotic twins. Psychiatrica Fennica 97–104, 1971

Windham GC, Bjerkedal LT: Malformations in twins and their siblings. Acta Genet Med Gemellol (Roma) 33:75–80, 1984

Section III

The Neurobiology of Schizophrenia

Traditional Methods and Emerging Technologies

The Neurobiology of Schizophrenia

Traditional Methods and Emerging Technologies

---◆---

Diseases in medicine are ultimately defined through identification of their underlying pathophysiology or etiology. For example, diabetes mellitus is defined as a disease caused by failure of insulin-producing cells in the pancreas, a pathophysiological explanation that gives diabetes mellitus a consistent and replicable explanation for its clinical manifestation, the appearance of increased glucose in the urine and blood. Subsequent studies have moved toward the identification of etiology, indicating that diabetes is a syndrome in which the clinical presentation and underlying pathophysiology can be due to a variety of mechanisms and causes, almost certainly including multiple genetic mechanisms as well as environmental influences.

Schizophrenia is often conceptualized as being similar to diabetes in pathophysiology and etiology, in that it is probably a heterogeneous group of disorders that are due to multiple mechanisms, which may be both genetic and environmental. Schizophrenia differs, however, in that it does not have a single identifiable pathophysiology. The search for the pathophysiology of schizophrenia has been long-standing, dating back to early work by Kraepelin, who initially defined the disorder. As pointed out in Chapter 7, however, the efforts to find a single consistent mechanism have met with failure.

Recent efforts to continue the search are reviewed in the two chapters in this section. Much of the emphasis of these efforts has been on studies that combine neuropathology and neurochemistry. One traditional approach is exemplified by Chapter 7, in which Dr. James A. Clardy and his colleagues describe the use of postmortem tissue to measure biochemical abnormalities in the brain and to search for specific regional abnormalities. A great deal of this work has focused on one particular neurotransmitter system—the dopamine system. Although it is clearly an oversimplification to perceive schizophrenia as a disease of dopamine dysregulation, nevertheless a substantial amount of evidence has been amassed that implicates dopamine abnormalities in the brain in schizophrenia.

The study of postmortem tissue has recently been supplemented by the application of neuroimaging techniques, as described in Chapter 8 by Dr. Göran Sedvall. These two approaches—the study of postmortem tissue and the use of in vivo neuroimaging—are best seen as complementary to one another. Each has particular strengths and weaknesses. A major strength of neuroimaging techniques is that they permit the study of first-episode and never-medicated patients. These techniques can be used, therefore, to study the mechanisms of schizophrenia independently of artifacts that might be produced by either treatment or chronicity. As summarized by Dr. Sedvall, the use of neuroimaging techniques has suggested the possibility of various metabolic and neurochemical abnormalities in schizophrenia, but the results are far from definitive. The lack of definitive findings is not surprising, however, considering the relative newness of the techniques and the great complexity and probable heterogeneity of schizophrenia.

Chapter 7

Postmortem Neurochemical and Neuropathological Studies in Schizophrenia

James A. Clardy, M.D.
Thomas M. Hyde, M.D., Ph.D.
Joel E. Kleinman, M.D., Ph.D.

———◆———

In a field Dr. Fred Plum (1972) once described as "the graveyard of neuropathologists," the neuropathology of schizophrenia has enjoyed a renaissance during the last two decades. Increased interest has been due to improved in vivo neuroimaging and neurophysiologic techniques as well as advances in postmortem neurochemical studies. Findings in one subfield of neuropathology often have served as corroboration of or impetus for investigation in other research modalities.

In this chapter we focus on postmortem neurochemical and neuropathological changes in schizophrenia with an emphasis on replicated findings. Postmortem studies have proved useful and have several advantages as described by Bracha and Kleinman (1984). First, the studied material can be subjected to a level of neuroanatomical resolution unattainable with in vivo neuroimaging. Second, postmortem studies spare living subjects the rigors and potential danger of study interventions. Third, some of the variability inherent in clinical trials may be eliminated.

Although postmortem studies continue to multiply, their reproduc-

123

ibility and interpretation remain as controversial as findings from half a century ago. Some inconsistencies may be attributable to differences between laboratories in patient diagnosis, medical and drug status of subjects at time of death, postmortem interval, brain storage, tissue dissection, and neurochemical techniques (Bracha and Kleinman 1984; Perry and Perry 1983; Rossor 1984; Spokes 1980).

An increase in type II (D_2) dopamine receptors in the basal ganglia (including nucleus accumbens) of brains of patients with schizophrenia is the most replicable postmortem neurochemical finding to date. It is likely that the basal ganglia, limbic system, and their innervating areas play an important role in schizophrenia. Studies that emphasize developmental aspects, neurochemical organization, and anatomical relationships of specific brain regions seem to be most useful. In this chapter we consider neurochemical and neuropathological changes following a neuroanatomical construct.

Basal Ganglia

Constituents of the basal ganglia that will be discussed here include the caudate, the putamen, the globus pallidus, and the nucleus accumbens. As shown in Table 7–1, the most replicable finding in postmortem neurochemical studies is the increased number of D_2 receptors in the caudate and the putamen. The interpretation of this finding remains controversial.

When Creese et al. (1976) showed that the relative antipsychotic potencies of neuroleptics correlated directly with their in vitro D_2 receptor blocking activity, it was speculated that an increase in number (B_{max}) and/or increased affinity (decreased K_d) of D_2 receptors was primarily involved in the mediation of certain schizophrenic symptoms. Since then it has been shown in animal studies that chronic neuroleptic D_2 receptor blockade gives rise to a dopamine supersensitivity with a subsequent increase in D_2 receptor number (Clow et al. 1980; Murugaiah et al. 1984). Human studies confirm the same effect on D_2 receptor number in the striatum (Joyce et al. 1988; Mjorndal and Winblad 1986; Seeman et al. 1987). The possibility that the striatal D_2 receptor increase is a treatment artifact rather than an intrinsic or primary neuropathological change continues to be the subject of controversy.

There is a significant body of evidence suggesting that the striatal D_2 receptor increase is primary to schizophrenia. Several studies relying on small numbers of drug-naive subjects found an increase in D_2 receptor density (Joyce et al. 1988; Lee et al. 1978; F. Owen et al. 1978). At least one in vivo positron-emission tomography (PET) study showed D_2 receptors increased in the striatum (Wong et al. 1986). Another study found that the severity of positive symptoms correlated with the quantity of D_2 receptors (Crow et al. 1981). A bimodal distribution for D_2 receptors, thought to be unrelated to treatment, was found in another group of schizophrenic patients (Seeman et al., 1984, 1987). Two studies comparing long-term neuroleptic-treated nonschizophrenic and schizophrenic patients found similar results. Seeman et al. (1987) found that patients with Alzheimer's and patients with Huntington's disease subjected to long-term neuroleptic therapy had striatal D_2 receptor increases of 40% or less, whereas neuroleptic-treated schizophrenic patients had doubled

Table 7–1.   Number of D_2 receptors in the basal ganglia and limbic system

Study	Caudate	Putamen	Nucleus accumbens
Lee et al. 1978; Lee and Seeman 1980	+	+	+
F. Owen et al. 1978	+	+	+
Mackay et al. 1980	NC		NC
Reisine et al. 1980	+	+	+
Reynolds et al. 1980		NC	
Cross et al. 1981	+		
Kleinman et al. 1982	+		
Mackay et al. 1982	+		+
Cross et al. 1983	+		
Seeman et al. 1984, 1987	+	+	+
Pimoule et al. 1985		+	
Mita et al. 1986	+		
Mjorndal and Winblad 1986	+	+	
Toru et al. 1986		+	
Wong et al. 1986	+		
Farde et al. 1987, 1990	NC	NC	
Hess et al. 1987	+		
Joyce et al. 1988	+	+	+
Kornhuber et al. 1989		NC	
Martinot et al. 1990	NC	NC	

Note.   + = increase. NC = no change.

or tripled densities of D_2 receptors. In another study using neuroleptic-treated Huntington's disease and senile dementia patients as comparisons to neuroleptic-treated schizophrenic patients, Seeman et al. (1987) found D_2 receptors increased in drug-free schizophrenic patients and increased further in drug-treated schizophrenic patients. The Huntington's disease and senile dementia cases showed no D_2 receptor increase after neuroleptic therapy. Investigators in both studies found the magnitude of D_2 increase in the schizophrenic population to be higher than predicted by neuroleptic exposure alone.

Despite the aforementioned data, there is some evidence to suggest that increased D_2 receptors in schizophrenia represent treatment artifact. Mackay et al. (1980) reported normal densities of D_2 receptors in schizophrenic patients off neuroleptics for at least 1 month. Reynolds et al. (1980) found subnormal caudate D_2 receptors in neuroleptic-treated patients and in those off neuroleptics for 3 or more months. It should be noted that the Mackay et al. study measured absolute receptor densities at only about 20% of values measured by other investigators, suggesting receptor degradation, whereas the Reynolds et al. study had very high K_d values, probably indicating considerable residual neuroleptic, which may mask receptor density (B_{max}) (Seeman 1981). Kornhuber et al. (1987a) found that D_2 B_{max} values in postmortem putamen samples from schizophrenic subjects were only increased in their study in patients who received neuroleptic medication within a 3-month period before death, but the subjects in this study were unusually old at age of disease onset.

Two recent PET studies failed to demonstrate a difference in striatal D_2 receptor concentration. Martinot et al. (1990) used 12 drug-free patients and acknowledged that their method was limited in that it allowed only global determination in an anatomically and functionally heterogeneous area. In the other PET study, Farde et al. (1990) used 18 neuroleptic-naive patients with schizophrenia and found no significant difference in B_{max} or K_d values in the putamen or the caudate.

The correlation between an increase in D_2 receptor density and an increased degree of positive symptoms may simply be due to a need for more neuroleptics in response to these symptoms (Jaskiw and Kleinman 1989). In the study finding a bimodal distribution of receptors (Seeman et al. 1984), the vast majority of patients off medication for longer than 6 months had D_2 receptors in the normal range in the caudate and the putamen. This finding can be interpreted in several ways. The authors argue that the bimodal distribution is not a result of neuroleptics, because the K_d between the two groups does not differ. Although the argument suggests that neuroleptics at the time of death were no different in either group of schizophrenic patients, it does not rule out any differences in chronic usage. One interpretation is that the receptor increase is in response to medication. Another possibility would be that a patient with a primary increase in receptor density would have more symptoms and be less likely to tolerate a drug-free period, thus distorting the study (Jaskiw and Kleinman 1989). It should be noted, however, that a bimodal curve would still exist if all neuroleptic-free patients were removed.

There is a paucity of type I (D_1) receptor studies compared with D_2 studies. Most studies involving the human basal ganglia have not shown a change in D_1 receptor concentration in patients with schizophrenia versus control subjects (Carenzi et al. 1975; Cross et al. 1981; Joyce et al. 1988; Pimoule et al. 1985; Seeman et al. 1987). Studies have shown no alteration in cerebral receptor number for animals receiving chronic neuroleptics (Mackenzie and Zigmond 1985; Murugaiah et al. 1984; Porceddu et al. 1985). One human study found an increase in D_1 receptor responsiveness in schizophrenic brains as shown by enhanced dopamine function, believed to be the expression of an increased efficiency in the G/F protein coupling operative in linking D_1 recognition sites to adenylate cyclase (Memo et al. 1983). Another study found a decrease in the concentration of D_1 receptors in the caudate nucleus of schizophrenic patients (Hess et al. 1987). Neither of these human studies has been replicated.

There is little consensus concerning changes in the density or affinity states of other receptor types in the basal ganglia (Table 7–2). Isolated positive studies have not been replicated. Studies on neurotransmitters, neuromodulators, and their metabolites and enzymes of synthesis and degradation have yielded inconclusive data (Table 7–3) (for a review of enzymes, see Kleinman 1986). In schizophrenic brains, a serotonin increase in the putamen (Crow et al. 1979; Korpi et al. 1986) and globus pallidus (Farley et al. 1980; Korpi et al. 1986) seems less tenuous, but only one study (Farley et al. 1980) showed a serotonin metabolite, 5-hydroxyindoleacetic acid, increased in the same area.

One innovative study suggested that studies of catecholamine and indoleamine uptake by synaptosomes from appropriately handled postmortem brain tissue may provide information about their presynaptic state (Haberland and Hetey 1987a). These investigators found increases in dopamine and norepinephrine uptake in the caudate in schizophrenic versus control brains.

Early reports (Bird et al. 1977, 1979a, 1979b) of an increase in nucleus accumbens dopamine concentration in schizophrenia have generally not been replicated (Crow et al. 1979; Farley et al. 1978, 1980; Kleinman et al. 1982; Toru et al. 1982). In one study, Mackay et al. (1982) reported an increased concentration in the accumbens, especially with early onset cases, but felt that their findings might be entirely iatrogenic because one of their subgroups, patients off neuroleptics for 1 month or more, had concentrations of dopamine near control values. Consistent with this, no increase in dopamine metabolite concentrations has been found in the accumbens from brains of schizophrenic subjects (Bacopoulos et al. 1979; Crow et al. 1979; Farley et al. 1977; Kleinman et al. 1982; Toru et al. 1982) (see Table 7–4).

Increases in D_2 receptors in the accumbens of schizophrenic patients have been reported (Joyce et al. 1988; Lee et al. 1978, 1980; Mackay et al. 1982; F. Owen et al. 1978; Seeman et al. 1984), but the same considerations that apply to the other basal ganglia areas are germane here. Although animal study (Rupniak et al. 1985) suggests that chronic neuroleptic treatment does not cause an increase in dopamine receptors

Table 7–2.   Non-D_2 receptors in the basal ganglia in schizophrenia

Study	Findings
Reisine et al. 1980	Decreased ^{3}H-naloxone binding in caudate
F. Owen et al. 1981	No change in binding in caudate and putamen: ^{3}H-ADTN, 5-HT, LSD, QNB, GABA, diazepam
Kleinman et al. 1982	No change in caudate binding: ^{3}H-naloxone, WB 4101 (α receptors), dihydroalprenolol (β receptors), QNB (muscarinic receptors), GTP, diazepam
Ferrier et al. 1985	No change in CCK binding in the globus pallidus or putamen
F. Owen et al. 1985	No change in binding in caudate: ^{3}H-naloxone and ^{3}H-etorphine
Hanada et al. 1986	Increased ^{3}H-muscimol (GABA receptor) binding in caudate
Kornhuber et al. 1989	Increased MK-801 (N-methyl-D-aspartate receptor, PCP binding site, and probable glutamatergic site) in putamen

Note. QNB = 3-quinuclidinyl benzilate. GTP = guanosine triphosphate. ^{3}H-ADTN = 2-amino-6,7-dihydroxy-1,2,3,4-tetrahydronaphthalene. 5-HT = 5-hydroxytryptamine (serotonin). LSD = lysergic acid diethylamide. GABA = gamma-aminobutyric acid. CCK = cholecystokinin. PCP = phencyclidine.

Table 7–3.   Neurotransmitters in the basal ganglia in schizophrenia

Study	Findings
Bird et al. 1977, 1979a, 1979b	No change in dopamine in putamen or caudate
Crow et al. 1979	Increased dopamine in caudate; increased 5-HT in putamen
Joseph et al. 1979	No change in 5-HT or 5-HIAA in basal ganglia
Farley et al. 1980	Increased 5-HT and 5-HIAA in globus pallidus
Mackay et al. 1982	Increased dopamine in caudate
Toru et al. 1982	No change in dopamine and increased HVA in caudate and putamen
Kleinman et al. 1983	Decreased Met-enkephalin in caudate; no change in Met-enkephalin in putamen and globus pallidus
Davis et al. 1986	β-endorphin metabolism different in putamen
Korpi et al. 1986	Increased 5-HT in globus pallidus and putamen; no change in 5-HT in caudate or 5-HIAA in basal ganglia
Mann et al. 1986	No change in MAO-A or MAO-B kinetics
Haberland and Hetey 1987b	Increased dopamine and norepinephrine reuptake in caudate
Korpi et al. 1987	No change in caudate: GABA, taurine, gly-threonine, glutamate, aspartate, glutamine, tryptophan, alanine

Note.   5-HT = 5-hydroxytryptamine (serotonin). 5-HIAA = 5-hydroxyindoleacetic acid.
HVA = homovanillic acid. MAO = monoamine oxidase. GABA = gamma-aminobutyric
acid.

Table 7–4.   Catecholamines and metabolites in the nucleus accumbens in schizophrenia

Study	DA	DOPAC	HVA	MHPG	NE
Bird et al. 1977, 1979a, 1979b	+				NC
Farley et al. 1977, 1978, 1980	NC		NC		+
Bacopoulos et al. 1979			NC		
Crow et al. 1979	NC	NC	NC		NC
Kleinman et al. 1982	NC	NC	NC	+	+
Mackay et al. 1982	+				
Toru et al. 1982	NC	NC	NC		

Note.   DA = dopamine. DOPAC = dihydroxyphenylacetic acid. HVA = homovanillic acid.
MHPG = 3-methoxy-4-hydroxyphenylglycol. NE = norepinephrine. + = increased. NC = no
change.

in the accumbens, long-term effects of neuroleptics on human receptors remain to be determined.

Farley et al. (1978) and Kleinman et al. (1982) reported increased norepinephrine levels in the accumbens of chronic paranoid schizophrenic patients; in the latter study an increase in the major norepinephrine metabolite, 3-methoxy-4-hydroxyphenylglycol, was also found. Norepinephrine increases in the accumbens were not found in two studies (Bird et al. 1979a, 1979b) that included patients with a variety of schizophrenic subtypes, not just the chronic paranoid type. Kleinman et al. (1982) argued that, in light of normal levels of norepinephrine in the accumbens of chronic undifferentiated patients and other psychotic neuroleptic-treated control subjects, the increase in chronic paranoid schizophrenia is less likely to be an artifact of treatment. An increase of norepinephrine and dopamine but not serotonin uptake by a synaptosomal homogenate made from postmortem nucleus accumbens tissue has also been reported (Haberland and Hetey 1987b). Increased uptake may reflect increased presynaptic activity in the norepinephrine- and dopamine-containing neurons projecting to the nucleus accumbens (Jaskiw and Kleinman 1989). Studies of other binding sites, enzymes, and neurotransmitters and their metabolites in the accumbens have so far been mostly negative (Cross et al. 1979; Farley et al. 1980; Iversen et al. 1979; Kleinman et al. 1985; Korpi et al. 1986; Perry et al. 1979) (for a review, see Kleinman 1986).

Classic neuropathological studies of the basal ganglia in schizophrenia have produced few significant findings. Neuronal loss was reported in the globus pallidus (Hopf 1952; Vogt and Vogt 1952), but this finding has not been replicated (Arendt et al. 1983). Bogerts et al. (1985) found a decrease in the volume of the globus pallidus interna in a morphometric study of brains from the Vogt Institute in Düsseldorf, Germany. The nucleus accumbens, which acts as an interface between the limbic system and the basal ganglia, may have decreased volume in patients with schizophrenia (Pakkenberg 1987). A prior study found no differences in the volume of the accumbems between schizophrenic patients and control subjects (Bogerts et al. 1985). Dom et al. (1981) reported decreased neuronal size in the accumbens. Quantitative neuroimaging studies are not available for the accumbens. Bogerts et al. (1983) reported that the lateral zone of the substantia nigra had decreased volume without neuronal loss, suggestive of a loss of neuropil.

The value of these findings from neuropathological studies of the basal ganglia can only be ascertained by their independent replication. It should be noted that the brains in the Vogt collection are particularly valuable because they were collected before the advent of neuroleptic therapy, thereby eliminating the confounding effects of medications.

Limbic System

For the purpose of this review the following areas are considered as components of the limbic system: hypothalamus, amygdala, hippocampus, ventral septum, mammillary bodies, bed nucleus of the stria terminalis, and the olfactory area. Most studies have been confined to the first three structures.

Neurochemical investigations of the hypothalamus have produced markedly inconsistent results. For instance, in studies using schizophrenic tissue, Farley et al. (1980) reported increased serotonin concentration in the lateral hypothalamus, but Winbald et al. (1979) reported decreased concentration and Korpi et al. (1986) reported no change in concentration with respect to control subjects in the whole hypothalamus. A similar situation is found with studies of hypothalamic norepinephrine (Farley et al. 1978; Kleinman et al. 1982). Since the hypothalamus is an anatomically and neurochemically heterogeneous region, such inconsistencies are hardly surprising. Wiegant et al. (1988) showed that the hypothalamic concentration of α- and δ-endorphins was significantly higher in schizophrenic brains, suggesting abnormal metabolism of endorphins.

One group reported an increase in dopamine (Reynolds 1983; Reynolds and Czudek 1987) and in homovanillic acid (HVA) (Reynolds and Czudek 1987) in the left amygdala of schizophrenic patients. However, an earlier study found that dopamine levels in the central nucleus of the amygdala, which contains most amygdala dopamine, were not significantly different from those of control subjects (Bird et al. 1979b). In Bird et al.'s investigation, left and right amygdala from different patients were compared, increasing the risk of falsely negative findings.

Ferrier et al. (1983, 1985) reported that cholecystokinin and somatostatin concentrations were decreased in both the amygdala and hippocampus in an investigation of schizophrenic patients with a preponderance of negative symptoms. Some of these findings have not been replicated, perhaps because younger subjects with less negative symptomatology were studied (Kleinman et al. 1983; Nemeroff et al. 1983). A decrease in hippocampal cholecystokinin concentration and receptor density was found by one group in two different experiments (Farmery et al. 1985; Ferrier et al. 1985). In another hippocampal study, Kornhuber et al. (1989b) found the glutamate-related N-methyl-D-aspartate (NMDA) receptor-coupled ion channel to be enhanced in patients with schizophrenia, suggesting presynaptic dysfunction of the glutamate system as the source of this abnormality. Kerwin et al. (1988) found glutamate-related kainate binding to be reduced in the right hippocampus versus the left.

Other postmortem neurochemical findings from patients with schizophrenia include 1) increased dopamine in the anterior perforated substance (Bird et al. 1977, 1979b); 2) increased norepinephrine in the ventral septum, the mammillary bodies, and the bed nucleus of the stria terminalis (Farley et al. 1978); and 3) increased serotonin in the medial olfactory area (Farley et al. 1980). As is the case for many other findings, these have not been replicated and their relationship to neuroleptic exposure remains problematic.

In vitro neuropathological studies using postmortem tissue and in vivo studies relying on modern neuroimaging techniques have been unusually productive in the identification of abnormalities within the limbic system. Six independent groups of investigators reported structural abnormalities in the hippocampal region in postmortem studies (Altshuler et al. 1990; Arnold et al. 1991; Bogerts et al. 1985; Brown et al. 1986; Colter et al. 1987; Jakob and Beckmann 1986; Jeste and Lohr 1989). Remarkably, all morphometric studies of this region found abnormalities. In an additional refinement, Brown et al. (1986) suggested that the left parahippocampal gyrus is more diminished in size than the right. This laterality finding appears to be an artifact of the absence of a control group without known psychopathology; the inclusion of the latter suggests that the abnormalities are bilateral (Altshuler et al. 1990).

In living schizophrenic patients, quantitative abnormalities on magnetic resonance imaging (MRI) scans have been described in the mesial temporal lobe (DeLisi et al. 1988; Rossi et al. 1990; Suddath et al. 1989, 1990). In a study of monozygotic twins discordant for schizophrenia, the anterior hippocampus was smaller bilaterally in the ill twin in 14 of 15 pairs, suggesting that abnormalities in the hippocampus are an intrinsic feature of the neuropathology of schizophrenia (Suddath et al. 1990). Taken together, postmortem and in vivo neuroimaging data suggest that structural abnormalities of the hippocampus, parahippocampal gyrus, and entorhinal cortex may play a major role in the neurobiology of schizophrenia.

The microscopic pathology that might contribute to the macroscopic changes in the volume of the medial temporal lobe attributed to schizophrenia has come under great scrutiny. Disarray of the dendritic arborizations of hippocampal pyramidal cells was reported by Scheibel and Kovelman (1981); however, this finding was disputed by Christison et al. (1989). Jakob and Beckmann (1986, 1989) described cytoarchitectonic abnormalities in the entorhinal cortex, primarily within layer 2. They suggested that these abnormalities most likely represented a developmental lesion. Their finding was replicated in part by Arnold et al.(1991) and Falkai et al. (1988). Remarkably, gliosis, the neuropathological footprint of acquired injury to the adult central nervous system, has not been reported in the mesial temporal lobe (Christison et al. 1989; Falkai et al. 1988; Jakob and Beckmann 1986; Scheibel and Kovelman 1981). Active investigation in a number of laboratories should clarify the nature of the pathological changes in the hippocampal region.

Other parts of the limbic system may exhibit neuropathological abnormalities in schizophrenia. In vivo neuroimaging studies have suggested hypothalamic abnormalities. The third ventricle is enlarged in 80% of computed tomography (CT) studies of schizophrenic patients, as noted in the comprehensive review by Shelton and Weinberger (1986). The anterior hypothalamus surrounds the third ventricle, and tissue loss in this region might underlie the changes noted on neuroimaging studies. Traditional postmortem studies of the hypothalamus in schizophrenia have not been conclusive. J. R. Stevens (1982) reported prominent gliosis in the hypothalamus, but this has not been replicated. Lesch and Bogerts (1984) found an attenuation of the periventricular hypothalamic gray matter in brains from the Vogt collection, but this finding has not been replicated either. Clearly, there is a pressing need for additional research into these neuroanatomical regions in schizophrenia.

Cerebral Cortex

The relative size and concomitant complexity of the cerebral cortex, the frontal areas in particular, are perhaps the most distinguishing features of the human brain. Given that schizophrenia appears to be a uniquely human condition, the search for cerebral cortical pathology is understandable. Studies involving the cortex, especially specific areas of the frontal cortex, have revealed abnormalities in several neurotransmitter systems that modulate dopaminergic transmission. The most promising findings involve cholecystokinin, neurotensin, kainic acid, and glutamate. Positive findings in the cerebral cortex of schizophrenic patients are summarized in Table 7–5. Studies in the cortex of serotonin and its metabolites (Korpi et al. 1986; Winbald et al. 1979), uptake of norepinephrine or dopamine by homogenates of frontal cortical synaptosomes (Haberland and Hetey 1987b), LSD receptors (Bennett et al. 1979; Whitaker et al. 1981), amino acids (Perry and Hansen 1985), HVA

Table 7–5.   Positive findings in the cerebral cortex

Study	Findings
Bennett et al. 1979	Decreased ^{3}H-LSD (5-HT) binding in frontal cortex
Quirion et al. 1982	Increased neurotensin binding in frontal cortex
Ferrier et al. 1983, 1985	Decreased CCK in temporal cortex; no change in CCK binding in frontal cortex or parietal cortex
Nemeroff et al. 1983	Increased neurotensin in frontal cortex
Nishikawa et al. 1983	Increased kainic acid binding in frontal cortex
Reynolds et al. 1983	Nonsignificant increase in ^{3}H-ketanserin (5-HT2) binding in frontal cortex
Farmery et al. 1985	Decreased CCK binding in frontal cortex
Manberg et al. 1985	Decreased TRH and SRIF in frontal cortex (Brodmann area 12); decreased TRH in frontal cortex (Brodmann area 32)
Hanada et al. 1986	Increased ^{3}H-muscimol (GABA) binding in prefrontal cortex
Mann et al. 1986	No change in 5-HT in frontal cortex
Mita et al. 1986	Decreased ketanserin (5-HT2) binding in prefrontal cortex
Toru et al. 1986	Increased ^{3}H-kainic acid (glutamate receptor) binding in medial frontal cortex and eye movement area; increased ^{3}H-QNB (muscarinic) binding in medial frontal cortex
Deakin et al. 1989	Increased [^{3}H]kainic acid (glutamate receptor) binding in orbital frontal cortex; increased D-[^{3}H]aspartate binding to glutamatergic uptake sites in orbital frontal cortex
Kornhuber et al. 1989	Nonsignificant increase in [^{3}H]MK-801 (NMDA glutamate receptor) binding in frontal cortex

Note. 5-HT = 5-hydroxytryptamine (serotonin). CCK = cholecystokinin. TRH = thyrotropin-releasing hormone. SRIF = somatostatin. GABA = gamma-aminobutyric acid. QNB = 3-quinuclidinyl benzilate. NMDA = N-methyl-D-aspartate.

(Bacopoulos et al. 1979), and glutamic acid dehydrogenase (Cross et al. 1979; Perry et al. 1979) have been negative.

The effects of neuroleptics, the lack of replicated findings, and the unknown degree of specificity for schizophrenia complicate the interpretation of studies of cortical neurochemistry in schizophrenia. Perhaps newly evolving pathophysiologic techniques and in vivo neuroimaging will serve to guide neurochemical studies to more specific areas of the cortex for more meaningful studies.

Comparatively few neuroimaging and neuropathological findings have been reported in the neocortex. On MRI scans, the volume of the temporal lobe gray matter is reduced in patients with schizophrenia (Suddath et al. 1989). However, it is unclear how much of this change results from pathology within the hippocampal region as opposed to changes within the entire cortex of the temporal lobe. Extratemporally, there have been scattered and poorly replicated reports of cortical gray matter attenuation and decreased cell counts (Alzheimer 1897; Benes et al. 1986; Kirch and Weinberger 1986; Pakkenberg 1987; Vogt and Vogt 1952). In the frontal lobes, which have been implicated in the neurobiology of schizophrenia in neuropsychological and functional neuroimaging studies (Weinberger 1988), few abnormalities have been reported. Jakob and Beckmann (1989) found abnormal gyral patterns in the frontal lobes. Other investigators have reported reductions in neuronal number and density in the prefrontal areas of the frontal cortex (Benes and Bird 1987; Benes et al. 1986; Colon 1972). Microscopically, axonal thickening was noted in the cerebral cortex and adjacent white matter in a study of biopsy specimens (Tatesu 1964). The significance of this finding, as well as of other putative neuropathological abnormalities in the cerebral cortex, is unclear.

Brain Stem and Other Areas

The source of most catecholamine and indoleamine input to subcortical and cortical structures—the brain stem—has been relatively neglected in postmortem studies. An increase of D_2 receptors in substantia nigra (R. Owen et al. 1984), decreased serotonin in the medulla and mesencephalon (Winbald et al. 1979), and increased norepinephrine in the pons (Carlsson 1980) have been reported in schizophrenic subjects.

A report that gamma-aminobutyric acid (GABA) is decreased in the thalamus (Perry et al. 1979) was not corroborated independently (Cross et al. 1979). However, both groups did find normal thalamic glutamic acid dehydrogenase activity (for a review of enzymes, see Kleinman 1986). An increase in somatostatin in the lateral thalamus was reported by Ferrier et al. (1983). Cholecystokinin levels in the lateral and dorsomedial thalamus were unchanged (Ferrier et al. 1985). Oke et al. (1988) found an increase in dopamine-to-norepinephrine ratios in the thalamus, lending some support to the 6-hydroxydopamine theory of schizophrenia (Stein and Wise 1972).

Neuropathology studies in the brain stem and thalamus also are scant. Bogerts et al. (1983) reported that the ventral tegmental area of the midbrain, the source of dopamine afferents to the limbic system, contains smaller cells in schizophrenic patients compared with control subjects. Fisman (1975) reported glial nodules in the pons, but this finding was contested (Hankoff and Perress 1981). Gliosis in the midbrain periaqueductal gray matter is yet another inconsistent finding (Hempel and Treff 1959; J. R. Stevens 1982). Thalamic pathological studies are equally underrepresented. Dom et al. (1981) reported decreased small neurons in the posterior thalamus; Lesch and Bogerts (1984) described diminished volume in the central nucleus of the thalamus. The dorsomedial thalamus, which links the accumbens and hypothalamus to the prefrontal cortex, also may have diminished volume and neuronal numbers (Hempel and Treff 1959; Pakkenberg 1990). Additional studies are needed.

Discussion

A review of the literature reveals no shortage of positive findings in postmortem neurochemical and neuropathological studies of the brains from patients with schizophrenia. Unfortunately, most of these findings have not been replicated, with the exception of increased D_2 receptors in the striatum and nucleus accumbens. The interpretation of this finding is confounded by the role of neuroleptics in producing this increase.

The difficulties in the delineation of the neurochemical and neuropathological abnormalities in the brains of patients with schizophrenia may be attributed to the absence of a well-defined and specific neuroanatomical substrate for psychosis. Fortunately, in the last several years investigators have started to focus with reasonable precision on a subset of structures whose involvement in schizophrenia seems promising. For instance, MRI studies have implicated the anterior hippocampus and temporal cortex, showing their reduced size in schizophrenic patients (Bogerts et al. 1990; Falkai et al. 1988). Regional cerebral blood flow linked to specific neuropsychological tasks has implicated the dorsolateral prefrontal cortex in schizophrenia (Weinberger et al. 1986). Lastly, neuronal morphometry has confirmed abnormalities in the anterior hippocampal and parahippocampal gyrus in postmortem studies (Altshuler et al. 1990; Arnold et al. 1991; Brown et al. 1986; Colter et al. 1987; Jakob and Beckmann 1986; Jeste and Lohr 1989). The neurochemical correlates of these structural abnormalities are areas ripe for investigation that, it is to be hoped, will yield greater reproducibility and new treatments.

References

Altshuler LL, Casanova MF, Goldberg TE, et al: The hippocampus and parahippocampus in schizophrenic, suicide, and control brains. Arch Gen Psychiatry 47:1029–1034, 1990

Alzheimer A: Deitrage zur pathologiischen Anatomie der Hirnrinde und zur anatomischen Grundlage einiger psychosen. Monatsschrift fur Psychiatrie und Neurologie 2:82–119, 1897

Arendt T, Bigl Y, Arendt A, et al: Loss of neurons in the nucleus basalis of Meynert in Alzheimer's disease, paralysis agitans, and Korsakoff's disease. Acta Neuropathol (Berl) 61:101–108, 1983

Arnold SE, Hyman BT, Van Hosen GW: Some cytoarchitectural abnormalities of the entorhinal cortex in schizophrenia. Arch Gen Psychiatry 48:625–632, 1991

Bacopoulos NC, Spokes EG, Bird EO, et al: Antipsychotic drug action in schizophrenic patients: effect on cortical dopamine metabolism after long-term treatment. Science 205:1405–1407, 1979

Benes FM, Bird ED: An analysis of the arrangement of neurons in the cingulate cortex of schizophrenic. Arch Gen Psychiatry 44:608–616, 1987

Benes FM, Davidson J, Bird ED: Quantitative cytoarchitectural studies of the cerebral cortex of schizophrenics. Arch Gen Psychiatry 43:31–35, 1986

Bennett JP, Enna SJ, Bylund DB, et al: Neurotransmitter receptors in frontal cortex of schizophrenics. Arch Gen Psychiatry 36:927–934, 1979

Bird EO, Spokes EG, Barnes J, et al: Increased brain dopamine and reduced glutamic acid decarboxylase and choline acetyltransferase activity in schizophrenia and related psychoses. Lancet 2:1157–1159, 1977

Bird EO, Spokes EGS, Iversen LL: Brain norepinephrine and dopamine in schizophrenia. Science 204:93–94, 1979a

Bird EO, Spokes EGS, Iversen LL: Increased dopamine concentration in limbic areas of brain from patients dying with schizophrenia. Brain 102:347–360, 1979b

Bogerts B, Hantsch J, Herzer M: A morphometric study of the dopamine-containing cell groups in the mesencephalon of normals, Parkinson patients, and schizophrenic. Biol Psychiatry 18:951–959, 1983

Bogerts B, Meertz E, Schonfeld-Bausch R: Basal ganglia and limbic system pathology in schizophrenia. Arch Gen Psychiatry 42:784–791, 1985

Bogerts B, Ashtari M, Degreef G, et al: Reduced temporal limbic structure volumes on magnetic resonance images in first episode schizophrenia. Psychiatry Research 35:1–13, 1990

Bracha HS, Kleinman JE: Postmortem studies in psychiatry. Psychiatr Clin North Am 7:473–485, 1984

Brown R, Colter N, Corsellis JAN, et al: Postmortem evidence of structural brain changes in schizophrenia. Arch Gen Psychiatry 43:36–42, 1986

Carenzi A, Gillin JC, Guidotti A, et al: Dopamine-sensitive adenylyl cyclase in human caudate nucleus: a study in control subjects and schizophrenic patients. Arch Gen Psychiatry 32:1056–1059, 1975

Carlsson A: The impact of catecholamine research in medical science and practice, in Catecholamines: Basic and Clinical Frontiers. Edited by Usdin E, Kopin I, Barchas JD. New York, Pergamon, 1980, pp 4–19

Christison GW, Casanova MF, Weinberger DR, et al: A quantitative investigation of hippocampal pyramidal cell size, shape, and variability of orientation in schizophrenia. Arch Gen Psychiatry 46:1027–1032, 1989

Clow A, Theodorou A, Jenner P, et al: A comparison of striatal and mesolimbic dopamine function in the rat during 6-month trifluoperazine administration. Psychopharmacology (Berl) 69:227–233, 1980

Colon EJ: Quantitative cytoarchitectonic of the human cerebral cortex in schizophrenic dementia. Acta Neuropathol (Berl) 20:1–10, 1972

Colter N, Battal S, Crow TJ, et al: White matter reduction in the parahippocampal gyrus of patients with schizophrenia (letter). Arch Gen Psychiatry 44:1023, 1987

Creese I, Burt DR, Snyder SH: Dopamine receptor binding predicts clinical and pharmacological potencies of antischizophrenic drugs. Science 192:481–483, 1976

Cross AJ, Crow TJ, Owen F: Gamma-aminobutyric acid in the brain in schizophrenia (letter). Lancet 1:560–561, 1979

Cross AJ, Crow TJ, Owen F: 3H-flupenthixol binding in postmortem brains of schizophrenics: evidence for a selective increase in dopamine D2 receptors. Psychopharmacology (Berl) 74:122–124, 1981

Cross AJ, Crow TJ, Ferrier IN, et al: Dopamine receptor changes in schizophrenia in relation to the disease process and movement disorder. J Neural Transm Suppl 18:265–272, 1983

Crow TJ, Baker HF, Cross AJ, et al: Monoamine mechanisms in chronic schizophrenia: postmortem neurochemical findings. Br J Psychiatry 132:249–256, 1979

Crow TJ, Owen F, Cross AJ, et al: Neurotransmitter enzymes and receptors in postmortem brain in schizophrenia: evidence that an increase in D2 dopamine receptors is associated with the Type I syndrome, in Transmitter Biochemistry of Human Brain Tissue. Edited by Riederer P, Usdin E. London, Macmillan, 1981, pp 85–96

Davis TP, Culling-Berglund AJ, Schoemaker H: Specific regional differences of in vitro B-endorphin metabolism in schizophrenics. Life Sci 39:2601–2609, 1986

Deakin JFW, Slater P, Simpson MDC, et al: Frontal cortical and left temporal glutamatergic dysfunction in schizophrenia. J Neurochem 52:1781–1786, 1989

DeLisi LE, Dauphinais ID, Gershon ES: Perinatal complications and reduced size of brain limbic structures in familial schizophrenia. Schizophr Bull 14:185–191, 1988

Dom R, De Saedeleer J, Bogerts J, et al: Quantitative cytometric analysis of basal ganglia in catatonic schizophrenics, in Biological Psychiatry. Edited by Perris C, Struwe G, Jansson B. New York, Elsevier, 1981, pp 723–726

Falkai P, Bogerts B, Rozumek M: Limbic pathology in schizophrenia: the entorhinal region—a morphometric study. Biol Psychiatry 24:515–521, 1988

Farde L, Wiesel F-A, Hall H, et al: No D2 receptor increase in PET study of schizophrenia. Arch Gen Psychiatry 44:671–672, 1987

Farde L, Wiesel F-A, Stone-Elander S, et al: D2 dopamine receptors in neuroleptic-naive schizophrenic patients. Arch Gen Psychiatry 47:213–219, 1990

Farley IJ, Price KS, Hornykiewicz O: Dopamine in the limbic regions of the human brain normal and abnormal. Adv Biochem Psychopharmacol 16:57–64, 1977

Farley IJ, Price KS, McCullough E, et al: Norepinephrine in chronic paranoid schizophrenia above-normal levels in limbic forebrain. Science 200:456–458, 1978

Farley IJ, Shannak KS, Hornykiewicz O: Brain monoamine changes in chronic paranoid schizophrenia and their possible relation to increased dopamine receptor sensitivity, in Receptors for Neurotransmitters and Peptide Hormones. Edited by Pepeu G, Kuhar MJ, Enna SJ. New York, Raven, 1980, pp 427–433

Farmery SM, Owen F, Poulter M, et al: Reduced high affinity cholecystokinin binding in hippocampus and frontal cortex of schizophrenia patients. Life Sci 36:472–478, 1985

Ferrier IN, Roberts GW, Crow TJ, et al: Reduced cholecystokinin-like and somatostatin-like immunoreactivity in limbic lobe is associated with negative symptoms in schizophrenia. Life Sci 33:475–482, 1983

Ferrier IN, Crow TJ, Farmery SM, et al: Reduced cholecystokinin levels in the limbic lobe in schizophrenia a marker for pathology underlying the defect state? Ann N Y Acad Sci 448:495–506, 1985

Fisman M: The brain stem in psychosis. Br J Psychiatry 126:414–422, 1975

Haberland N, Hetey L: Studies in postmortem dopamine uptake, I: kinetic characterization of the synaptosomal dopamine uptake in rat and human brain after postmortem storage and cryopreservation—comparison with noradrenaline and serotonin uptake. J Neural Transm 68:289–301, 1987a

Haberland N, Hetey L: Studies in postmortem dopamine uptake, II: alterations of the synaptosomal catecholamine uptake in postmortem brain regions in schizophrenia. J Neural Transm 68:303–313, 1987b

Hanada S, Mita T, Nishino N, et al: [3H]muscimol binding in autopsied brains of chronic schizophrenics. Life Sci 40:259–266, 1986

Hankoff LD, Perress NS: Neuropathology of the brain stem in psychiatric disorder. Biol Psychiatry 16:945–952, 1981

Hempel KJ, Treff WM: Uber normale Lucken und pathologische Luchkenbildung in einem subkortikalen Prisma (mediodoraler Thalamuskern). Beitr Path Anat 121:288–300, 1959

Hess EJ, Bracha HS, Kleinman JE, et al: Dopamine receptor subtype imbalance in schizophrenia. Life Sci 40:1487–1497, 1987

Hopf A: Uber histopathologische Veranderungen im Pallidum und Striatum bei Schizophrenie, in Proceedings of the First International Congress on Neuropathology, Vol 3. Turin, Italy, Rosenberg and Sellier, 1952, pp 629–635

Iversen LL, Bird E, Spokes E, et al: Agonist specificity of GABA binding sites in human brain and GABA in Huntington's disease and schizophrenia, in GABA-Neurotransmitters: Pharmacochemical, Biochemical and Pharmacological Aspects. Edited by Krogsgaard-Larsen P, Scheel-Kruger J, Kofod H. New York, Academic Press, 1979, pp 179–190

Jakob H, Beckmann H: Prenatal developmental disturbances in the limbic allcortex in schizophrenics. J Neural Transm 65:303–326, 1986

Jakob H, Beckmann H: Gross and histological criteria for developmental disorders in brains of schizophrenics. J R Soc Med 82:466–469, 1989

Jaskiw G, Kleinman JE: Postmortem neurochemistry studies in schizophrenia, in Schizophrenia: Scientific Progress. Edited by Schulz SC, Tamminga CA. New York, Oxford University Press, 1989, pp 264–273

Jeste DV, Lohr JB: Hippocampal pathological findings in schizophrenia: a morphometric study. Arch Gen Psychiatry 46:1019–1024, 1989

Joseph MH, Baker HF, Crow TJ, et al: Brain tryptophan metabolism in schizophrenia: a post mortem study of metabolites on the serotonin and kynurenine pathways in schizophrenic and control subjects. Psychopharmacology (Berl) 62:279–285, 1979

Joyce JN, Lexow N, Bird E, et al: Organization of dopamine D1 and D2 receptors in human striatum: receptor autoradiographic studies in Huntington's disease and schizophrenia. Synapse 2:546–557, 1988

Kerwin RW, Patel S, Meldrum BS, et al: Asymmetrical loss of glutamate receptor subtype in left hippocampus in schizophrenia. Lancet 1:583–584, 1988

Kirch DG, Weinberger DR: Anatomical neuropathology in schizophrenia: postmortem findings, in Handbook of Schizophrenia, Vol 1: The Neurology of Schizophrenia. Edited by Nasrallah HA, Weinberger DR. Amsterdam, Elsevier, 1986, pp 325–348

Kleinman JE: Postmortem neurochemistry observations in schizophrenia, in Handbook of Schizophrenia, Vol 1: The Neurology of Schizophrenia. Edited by Nasrallah HA, Weinberger DR. Amsterdam, Elsevier, 1986, pp 349–360

Kleinman J, Karoum F, Rosenblatt JE, et al: Postmortem neurochemical studies in chronic schizophrenia, in Biological Markers in Psychiatry and Neurology. Edited by Usdin E, Hanin I. New York, Pergamon, 1982

Kleinman JE, Iadarola M, Govoni S, et al: Postmortem measurements of neuropeptides in human brain. Psychopharmacol Bull 19:375–379, 1983

Kleinman JE, Hong J, Iadarola M, et al: Neuropeptides in human brains: postmortem studies. Progress in Neuro-Psychopharmacology 9:91–95, 1985

Kornhuber J, Riederer P, Reynolds GP, et al: 3H-spiperone binding sites in postmortem brains from schizophrenic patients: relationship to neuroleptic drug treatment, abnormal movements, and positive symptoms. Journal of Neural Transmission 75:1–10, 1989a

Kornhuber J, Mack-Burkhardt F, Riederer P, et al: [3H]MK-801 binding sites in postmortem brain regions of schizophrenic patients. Journal of Neural Transmission 77:231–236, 1989b

Korpi ER, Kleinman JE, Goodman SI, et al: Serotonin and 5-hydroxyindoleacetic acid concentrations in different brain regions of suicide victims: comparison in chronic schizophrenic patients with suicides as cause of death. Arch Gen Psychiatry 43:594–600, 1986

Korpi ER, Kleinman JE, Goodman SI, et al: Neurotransmitter amino acids in postmortem brains of chronic schizophrenic patients. Psychiatry Res 22:291–301, 1987

Lee T, Seeman P: Elevation of brain neuroleptic/dopamine receptors in schizophrenia. Am J Psychiatry 137:191–197, 1980

Lee T, Seeman P, Tourtelotte WW, et al: Binding of 3H-neuroleptics and 3H-apomorphine in schizophrenic brains. Nature 274:897–900, 1978

Lesch A, Bogerts B: The diencephalon in schizophrenia: evidence of reduced thickness of the periventricular grey matter. Eur Arch Psychiatry Neurol Sci 234:212–219, 1984

Mackay AVP, Bird O, Bird ED, et al: Dopamine receptors and schizophrenia: drug effect or illness? Lancet 2:915–916, 1980

Mackay AP, Iversen LL, Rossor M, et al: Increased brain dopamine and dopamine receptors in schizophrenia. Arch Gen Psychiatry 39:991–997, 1982

Mackenzie RG, Zigmond MJ: Chronic neuroleptic treatment increases D2 but not D1 receptors in rat striatum. Eur J Pharmacol 113:159–165, 1985

Manberg PJ, Nemeroff CB, Bisette G, et al: Neuropeptides in CSF and postmortem brain tissue of normal controls and schizophrenics and Huntington choreics. Prog Neuropsychopharmacol Biol Psychiatry 9:97–108, 1985

Mann JJ, Kaplan RD, Bird ED: Elevated postmortem monoamine oxidase B activity in the caudate nucleus in Huntington's disease compared to schizophrenics and controls. Journal of Neural Transmission 65:277–283, 1986

Martinot J, Peron-Magnan P, Huret J, et al: Striatal D2 dopamine receptors assessed with positron emission tomography and [76Br]bromospiperone in untreated schizophrenic patients. Am J Psychiatry 147:44–50, 1990

Memo M, Kleinman JE, Hanbauer I: Coupling of dopamine D1 recognition sites with adenylate cyclase in nuclei accumbens and caudatus of schizophrenics. Science 221:1304–1307, 1983

Mita T, Hanada S, Nishino N, et al: Decreased serotonin S2 and increased dopamine D2 receptors in chronic schizophrenics. Biol Psychiatry 21:1407–1414, 1986

Mjorndal T, Winblad B: Alteration of dopamine receptors in the caudate nucleus and the putamen in schizophrenic brain. Medical Biology 64:351–354, 1986

Murugaiah K, Fleminger S, Hall MD, et al: Alterations in different populations of striatal dopamine receptors produced by 18 months continuous administration of cis- or trans-flupenthixol to rats. Neuropharmacology 23:599–609, 1984

Nemeroff CB, Youngblood WW, Manberg PJ, et al: Regional brain concentrations of neuropeptides in Huntington's chorea and schizophrenia. Science 221:972–975, 1983

Nishikawa T, Takashima M, Toru M: Increased [3H]kainic acid binding in the prefrontal cortex in schizophrenia. Neurosci Lett 40:245–250, 1983

Oke AF, Adams RN, Winblad B, et al: Elevated dopamine/norepinephrine ratios in thalami of schizophrenic brains. Biol Psychiatry 24:79–82, 1988

Owen F, Cross AJ, Crow TJ, et al: Increased dopamine-receptor sensitivity in schizophrenia. Lancet 2:223–225, 1978

Owen F, Cross AJ, Crow TJ, et al: Neurotransmitter receptors in brain in schizophrenia. Acta Psychiatr Scand Suppl 291:20–28, 1981

Owen F, Bourne RC, Poulter M, et al: Tritiated etorphine and naloxone binding to opioid receptors in caudate nucleus in schizophrenia. Br J Psychiatry 146:507–509, 1985

Owen R, Owen F, Poulter M, et al: Dopamine D2 receptors in substantia nigra in schizophrenia. Brain Res 299:153–154, 1984

Pakkenberg B: Postmortem study of chronic schizophrenic brains. Br J Psychiatry 151:744–752, 1987

Pakkenberg B: Pronounced reduction of total neuron number in mediodorsal thalamic nucleus and nucleus accumbens in schizophrenics. Arch Gen Psychiatry 47:1023–1028, 1990

Perry T, Hansen S: Interconversion of serine and glycine is normal in psychiatric patients. Psychiatry Res 15:109–113, 1985

Perry EK, Perry RH: Human brain neurochemistry: some postmortem problems. Life Sci 3:1733–1743, 1983

Perry TL, Kish SJ, Buchanan J, et al: Gamma aminobutyric-acid deficiency in brain of schizophrenic patients. Lancet 1:237–239, 1979

Pimoule C, Shoemaker H, Reynolds GP, et al: [3H]SCH 23390 labeled D1 dopamine receptors are unchanged in schizophrenia and Parkinson's disease. Eur J Pharmacol 114:235–237, 1985

Plum F: Prospects for research on schizophrenia, 3: neuropsychology, neuropathological findings. Neurosciences Research Program Bulletin 10:384–388, 1972

Porceddu ML, Ongini E, Biggio G: [3H]SCH 23390 binding sites increase after chronic blockage of D1 dopamine receptors. Eur J Pharmacol 118:367–370, 1985

Quirion R, Larsen TA, Calne D, et al: Analysis of [3H]neurotensin receptors by computerized densitometry visualization of central and peripheral neurotensin receptors. Ann N Y Acad Sci 400:415–417, 1982

Reisine TD, Rossor M, Spokes E, et al: Opiate and neuroleptic receptor alterations in human schizophrenic brain tissue, in Receptors for Neurotransmitters and Peptide Hormones. Edited by Pepeu G, Kuhar MJ, Enna SJ. New York, Raven, 1980, pp 443–450

Reynolds G: Increased concentrations and lateral asymmetries of amygdala dopamine in schizophrenia. Nature 306:527–529, 1983

Reynolds GP, Czudek C: Neurochemical laterality of the limbic system in schizophrenia, in Cerebral Dynamics, Laterality and Psychopathology. Edited by Takahashi R, Flor-Henry P, Gruzelier J, et al. New York, Elsevier Science, 1987, pp 451–456

Reynolds GP, Reynolds LM, Riederer P, et al: Dopamine receptors and schizophrenia: drug effect or illness (letter)? Lancet 2:1251, 1980

Reynolds GP, Rossor MN, Iversen LL: Preliminary studies of human cortical 5-HT2 receptors and their involvement in schizophrenia and neuroleptic drug action. J Neural Transm Suppl 18:273–277, 1983

Rossi A, Stratta P, D'Albenzio L, et al: Reduced temporal lobe areas in schizophrenia. Biol Psychiatry 27:61–68, 1990

Rossor M: Biological markers in mental disorders postmortem studies. J Psychiatr Res 18:457–465, 1984

Rupniak NMJ, Hall MD, Kelly E, et al: Mesolimbic dopamine function is not altered during continuous treatment of rats with typical or atypical neuroleptic drugs. J of Neural Transmission 62:249–266, 1985

Scheibel AB, Kovelman JA: Disorientation of the hippocampal pyramidal cell and its processes in the schizophrenic patient. Biol Psychiatry 16:101–102, 1981

Seeman P: Dopamine receptors in postmortem schizophrenia brains (letter). Lancet 1:1103, 1981

Seeman P, Ulpian C, Bergeron C, et al: Bimodal distribution of dopamine receptor densities in brains of schizophrenics. Science 225:728–731, 1984

Seeman P, Bzowej NH, Guan HC, et al: Human brain D1 and D2 dopamine receptors in schizophrenia, Alzheimer's, Parkinson's, and Huntington's diseases. Neuropsychopharmacology 1:5–15, 1987

Shelton RC, Weinberger DR: X-ray computerized tomography studies in schizophrenia: a review and synthesis, in Handbook of Schizophrenia, Vol 1: The Neurology of Schizophrenia. Edited by Nasrallah HA, Weinberger DR. Amsterdam, Elsevier, 1986, pp 207–250

Spokes EGS: Neurochemical alterations in Huntington's chorea: a study of postmortem human tissue. Brain 103:179–210, 1980

Stein W, Wise CD: Possible etiology of schizophrenia: progressive damage to the noradrenergic reward system by endogenous 6-hydroxydopamine. Res Publ Assoc Res Nerv Ment Dis 50:298–314, 1972

Stevens CD, Altshuler LL, Bogerts B, et al: Quantitative study of gliosis in schizophrenia and Huntington's chorea. Biol Psychiatry 24:697–700, 1988

Stevens JR: Neuropathology of schizophrenia. Arch Gen Psychiatry 39:1131–1139, 1982

Suddath RL, Casanova MF, Goldberg TE, et al: Temporal lobe pathology in schizophrenia: a quantitative magnetic resonance imaging study. Am J Psychiatry 146:464–472, 1989

Suddath RL, Christison GW, Torrey EF, et al: Anatomical abnormalities in the brains of monozygotic twins discordant for schizophrenia. N Engl J Med 322:789–794, 1990

Tatesu S: A contribution to the morphological background of schizophrenia: with special reference to the findings in the telencephalon. Acta Neuropathol (Berl) 3:558–571, 1964

Toru M, Nishikawa T, Matag N: Dopamine metabolism increases in postmortem schizophrenic basal ganglia. Journal of Neural Transmission 54:181–191, 1982

Toru M, Watanabe S, Nishikawa T, et al: Neurotransmitter receptors in postmortem schizophrenic brains, in Recent Research on Neurotransmitter Receptors. Edited by Yoshida H. Tokyo, Excerpta Medica, 1986, pp 94–103

Vogt C, Vogt O: Alterations anatomiques de la schizophrenie et d'autres psychoses dites functionelles, in Proceedings of the First International Congress of Neuropathology, Vol 1. Turin, Italy, Rosenberg and Sellier, 1952, pp 515–532

Weinberger DR: Schizophrenia and the frontal lobe. Trends Neurosci 11:367–370, 1988

Weinberger DR, Berman KF, Zec RF: Physiologic dysfunction of dorsolateral prefrontal cortex in schizophrenia, I: regional cerebral blood flow evidence. Arch Gen Psychiatry 43:114–124, 1986

Whitaker PM, Crow TJ, Ferrier IN: Tritiated LSD binding in frontal cortex in schizophrenia. Arch Gen Psychiatry 38:278–280, 1981

Wiegant VM, Verhoef CJ, Burbach JPH, et al: Increased concentration of alpha and gamma endorphine in postmortem hypothalamic tissue of schizophrenic patients. Life Sci 42:1733–1742, 1988

Winbald B, Bucht G, Gottfries CG, et al: Monoamines and monoamine metabolites in brains from demented schizophrenics. Acta Psychiatr Scand 60:17–28, 1979

Wong DF, Wagner HN, Tune LE, et al: Positron emission tomography reveals elevated D2 dopamine receptors in drug-naive schizophrenics. Science 234:1558–1563, 1986

Chapter 8

Positron-Emission Tomography as a Metabolic and Neurochemical Probe

Göran Sedvall, M.D., Ph.D.

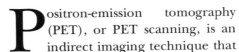

P ositron-emission tomography (PET), or PET scanning, is an indirect imaging technique that allows the analysis of the time course for distribution of intravenously administered labeled molecules within the living human brain. Such labeled molecules, called "tracers," can be designed to behave in biological systems in a way that reflects functional or biochemical aspects of dynamic brain events. Tracer molecules for glucose metabolism, oxygen consumption, blood flow, blood volume, and neurotransmitter functions as receptor characteristics have been developed.

The tracer molecules are tagged by a positron emitter, a specific type of radioactive isotope. These isotopes have the advantage of being short-lived. Upon disintegration such isotopes emit positrons, which when colliding with and annihilating electrons in the tissue cause the release of

Research described in this article was supported by the Swedish Medical Research Council (03560), the National Institute of Mental Health (41205, 44814), the Bank of Sweden Tercentenary Foundation (0427), and the Karolinska Institute.

gamma radiation of an intensity and type that allows external detection of the radiation. When a positron and an electron are annihilated, two gamma rays are released at 180° from each other. Therefore, two gamma ray–sensitive scintillation detectors placed diametrically in a ring around the head, when coincidence coupled, supply information concerning a line within the brain where the annihilation of the two particles has occurred. By feeding the information from a great number of such coincidence-coupled pairs of scintillation detectors into a computer, images of radioactivity can be constructed using mathematical techniques that allow the quantitative measurement and visualization of regional radioactivity in the brain during a defined time period. Using this procedure the labeled tracer molecules can be detected and followed in time by sampling radioactivity in small brain areas at preselected time windows after administration of the labeled molecule.

The first PET cameras developed and used in clinical neuropsychiatric research before 1980 had a resolution of approximately 15 mm. The present generation of cameras developed in 1990 have a resolution in one or all of the three planes on the order of 3–6 mm.

The first clinical studies of schizophrenic patients using PET were initiated in the early 1980s. During the past decade several studies have specifically addressed the question of brain functioning in schizophrenia. Two major areas have been explored: 1) regional brain energy metabolism in schizophrenia and 2) the analysis of dopamine receptor functions in schizophrenia.

Regional Brain Energy Metabolism in Schizophrenia

Most of the PET studies in schizophrenic patients have used 2-deoxyglucose labeled with fluorine-18 or carbon-11. In addition to these tracers, glucose labeled with ^{11}C in different positions has been used as a tool for PET research. Several but not all of the groups conducting this research found reduced rates of glucose metabolism in neocortical and central brain regions (for a review, see Wiesel 1989). The variance of metabolic rates was generally higher in the patients than in the control subjects. Patients with negative symptoms and a chronic course of the disease tended to show a more reduced metabolism. There was no consistent evidence of asymmetry or relationship to evidence of brain atrophy. Most of the studies were done in schizophrenic patients who had previously been drug treated but who had been off drugs for several weeks before the PET studies were performed. In one study where only drug-naive patients were examined, the results did not differ conspicuously from the studies where mixed drug-naive and drug-treated patients were examined (Cleghorn et al. 1989). Although the reduction of metabolism in the schizophrenic patients was significant in several regions, in most of the studies, the mean reduction was never greater than about 20% as compared with the control subjects, and in all studies there was considerable overlap of the metabolic rates between the patients and the control subjects.

PET studies of regional brain energy metabolism during activation of specific functional systems (i.e., during stimulation or the execution of specific psychological or psychometric tests) have also been performed. Using such a paradigm, Cohen et al. (1987) compared healthy control subjects with schizophrenic patients. They found reduced metabolic rates in the middle prefrontal cortex during the performance of auditory discrimination. Gur et al. (1989) found evidence that a higher left- relative to right-hemispheric cortical cerebral metabolic rate was associated with greater severity of symptoms specific to schizophrenia. Early et al. (1987), measuring blood flow with PET, found an abnormally high flow in the left globus pallidus of patients with schizophrenia.

In general it can be stated that the findings from PET studies of regional glucose metabolism are not consistent, and none of the findings were replicated. However, several of the studies gave results that allowed the formulation of a specific hypothesis regarding an aberration of regional energy metabolism in the brain of schizophrenic patients. These hypotheses can be summarized as follows:

1. Reduced frontal or prefrontal metabolism
2. General reduction of metabolism
3. Left relative hypermetabolism
4. Left relative temporal lobe hypermetabolism
5. Left globus pallidus abnormality

Future high-resolution PET scan studies in schizophrenia should focus on the explicit examination of each of these hypotheses in patient and control populations and should include drug-naive young patients. At least 20 individuals in each subject group should be examined with magnetic resonance imaging (MRI) verification of the anatomical structures in which the metabolic rates are determined.

Regional Brain Glucose Metabolism During Neuroleptic Treatment

Several investigators measuring glucose metabolism with PET compared schizophrenic patients before and after a standardized neuroleptic drug treatment related to a positive therapeutic response with regard to the psychosis (Buchsbaum et al. 1987; Wik et al. 1989). These studies showed no or an inconsistent increase of metabolism in the basal ganglia or several regions of the brain after antipsychotic drug treatment. Thus the PET studies of brain energy metabolism performed so far have had a low potential of disclosing effects of antipsychotic drugs and accordingly have given few new leads as to the mechanism behind antipsychotic effects of drugs.

PET Studies of Dopamine Receptors in Schizophrenia

Because PET makes it possible to study the distribution of labeled compounds in living human subjects, this technique also allows the recording of in vivo ligand binding to neuroreceptors in the brain. In the 1980s a great number of ligands were developed and used in experimental work, both in vitro and in vivo, to examine the characteristics of receptors for the major monoaminergic transmitter amines. In schizophrenia research it is obvious that an analysis of dopamine receptor characteristics should be of interest. Such an analysis could make it possible to evaluate experimentally the dopamine hypothesis for the pathophysiology of schizophrenia.

Most interest has been related to the dopamine D_2 receptors, so PET research has focused on the development of ligands for this receptor. Three types of ligands have now been used in PET scan studies on D_2 receptors in schizophrenia (for a review, see Sedvall 1992): ^{11}C-N-methylspiperone, 76-bromospiperone, and ^{11}C-raclopride. Of these, ^{11}C-raclopride has the highest selectivity with regard to specific binding to D_2 receptors. On the other hand, ^{11}C-N-methylspiperone and 76-bromospiperone have higher affinities for D_2 receptors, but these ligands also have significant affinities for serotonin 5-HT$_2$ receptors as well as for other binding sites.

Four clinical studies have been reported using these three ligands in schizophrenic patients. Wong et al. (1986), studying drug-naive schizophrenic patients and using [11]C-*N*-methylspiperone, found a two- to three-fold elevation of the number of D_2 binding sites in the caudate and the putamen. Crawley et al. (1986) used 76-bromospiperone as the ligand in single photon emission computed tomography (SPECT) to study schizophrenic patients who had previously been treated with neuroleptic drugs. They found a slight elevation of the binding potential, that is, the radioactivity ratio of the D_2 receptor–rich caudate to the dopamine receptor–poor cerebellum. Martinot et al. (1990), using the same ligand as Crawley et al., found that patients with an acute schizophrenic disorder with positive symptoms tended to have an elevated binding potential, whereas patients with chronic schizophrenia had reduced binding potential. Farde et al. (1987), studying ^{11}C-raclopride binding in completely drug-naive young schizophrenic patients, found the number and distribution of D_2 receptors in the caudate and the putamen similar to that found in healthy control subjects. These authors used a procedure allowing the determination of the affinity for the D_2 receptors. The results indicated an affinity of the ligand for central D_2 receptors in the drug-naive schizophrenic patients similar to that seen in the control subjects (Figure 8–1).

It seems clear at present that only prospective studies where [11]C-*N*-methylspiperone and ^{11}C-raclopride are used in a similar setting to examine D_2 receptors in schizophrenic patients are required to definitely settle the question concerning whether there are significant alterations of D_2 receptors in the brains of schizophrenic patients. A detailed account of the quantitative procedures used for determining D_2 receptor characteristics in the PET studies described in this section is presented in my review (Sedvall 1992). This review also presents some of the clinical and experimental differences among the PET studies of dopamine receptors in schizophrenia.

PET Studies of Dopamine Receptors in Schizophrenic Patients Treated With Antipsychotic Drugs

Although so far PET has failed to demonstrate consistently a general alteration of D_2 receptor characteristics in schizophrenia, this technique has been most influential in disclosing for the first time how antipsychotic drug treatment affects dopamine receptor functions in the brains of living patients (Farde et al. 1986, 1988; Sedvall et al. 1986). This was first shown in a series of studies using ^{11}C-raclopride as the ligand for D_2 receptors and ^{11}C-Sch 23390 for D_1 receptors. In relation to conventional clinical treatment with antipsychotic drugs of all the different chemical categories, a substantial fraction of the D_2 receptors in the major basal ganglia were found to be occupied. This held true for conventional drugs as well as unconventional drugs such as clozapine. Whereas the conventional compounds induced a more than 65% occupancy of D_2 receptors, clozapine treatment in a conventional antipsychotic dose induced only a 40%–65% occupancy of the D_2 receptors, which may be related to the low tendency of this drug to induce extrapyramidal symptoms. The effect of the antipsychotic drugs was pharmacologically specific because such an effect was not induced by other types of psychoactive drugs such as the antidepressant nortriptyline and the 5-HT$_2$ antagonist ritanserin.

PET scanning with ^{11}C-raclopride also disclosed that the degree of D_2 receptor occupancy was high early in relation to treatment and that it was dose dependent (Farde et al. 1988). There was a curvilinear relationship between the degree of occupancy and the dose of the drug as well as its plasma concentration. The occupancy also disappeared upon withdrawal of the drugs with a time course that was related to the plasma half-life of the compounds. Thus it has been demonstrated in living patients that

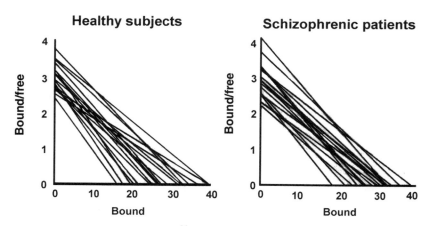

Figure 8–1. Scatchard plots for ^{11}C-raclopride binding to D_2 receptors in the putamen of healthy subjects ($n = 20$) and drug-naive schizophrenic patients ($n = 18$). The intercept of the lines with the abscissa indicates the maximal number of binding sites for D_2 receptors (B_{max}). The slope of the lines indicates the affinity for the D_2 receptors (K_d). *Source.* Data from L. Farde, F.-A. Wiesel, A.-L. Nordström, C. Halldin, and G. Sedvall, unpublished observations, March 1988.

there is a marked time difference between the points for both appearance and disappearance of dopamine receptor blockade and the time points for appearance and disappearance of the clinical antipsychotic effect that showed marked latencies. It has also been shown that so-called neuroleptic-resistant patients in general have about the same degree of D_2 receptor blockade as patients who respond to the treatment (Wolkin et al. 1989). It is accordingly evident that neuroleptic resistance must be related to factors other than a low D_2 receptor blockade. In all probability individual pathophysiological variance of brain function in schizophrenia is a major source of variance for neuroleptic response.

PET studies on D_1 receptors using the ligand ^{11}C-SCH 23390 demonstrated that some of the antipsychotic drugs, besides having an effect on D_2 receptors, also profoundly affect and block the D_1 receptors (Farde et al. 1989). This effect was particularly marked for the atypical antipsychotic drug clozapine, which was found to exhibit about the same degree of D_1 as D_2 receptor blockade when given in clinical doses to schizophrenic patients.

Summary

Since the early 1980s the PET technique has been applied in several studies to examine brain energy metabolism and dopamine receptor functions in schizophrenia. So far these studies have failed to demonstrate a consistent pattern of alterations of regional energy metabolism in the human brain in relation to schizophrenic symptoms. Neither have they been able to demonstrate consistently a general alteration of D_2 receptor characteristics. Studies of energy metabolism also have failed to disclose any reproducible effect of antipsychotic drug treatment.

On the other hand, PET measurements of dopamine receptor functions using ligands of antagonistic type for D_2 and D_1 receptors have demonstrated powerful and specific effects of antipsychotic drugs. In the studies cited in this chapter, conventional antipsychotic compounds all induced a marked occupancy of the population of D_2 receptors in the basal ganglia in relation to administration of clinical doses. The unconventional drug clozapine tended to have a lesser effect than the conventional drugs in this regard. Clozapine also induced a significant occupancy of D_1 receptors, whereas the conventional drugs induced a lesser effect on this receptor subtype. These results may be interpreted to indicate that blockade of D_2 as well as D_1 receptors may have beneficial effects on psychotic symptoms.

The implementation of new high-resolution PET cameras and the further development and application of more specific tracers for dopamine receptor subtypes and other transmitter mechanisms such as the serotonin 5-HT$_2$ receptor, the sigma opiate receptor, and benzodiazepine receptors will in all probability provide powerful tools for the further search for fundamental alterations of brain functions in schizophrenia.

References

Buchsbaum MS, Wu JC, DeLisi LE, et al: Positron emission tomography studies of basal ganglia and somatosensory cortex neuroleptic drug effects: differences between controls and schizophrenic patients. Biol Psychiatry 22:479–494, 1987

Cleghorn JM, Garnett ES, Nahmias C, et al: Increased frontal and reduced parietal glucose metabolism in acute untreated schizophrenia. Psychiatry Res 28:119–133, 1989

Cohen RM, Semple WE, Gross M, et al: Dysfunction in a prefrontal substrate of sustained attention in schizophrenia. Life Sci 40:2031–2039, 1987

Crawley CW, Crow TJ, Johnstone EC, et al: Uptake of [77]Br-spiperone in the striata of schizophrenic patients and controls. Nucl Med Commun 7:599–607, 1986

Early TS, Reiman EM, Raichle ME, et al: Left globus pallidus abnormality in never-medicated patients with schizophrenia. Proc Natl Acad Sci U S A 84:561–563, 1987

Farde L, Hall H, Ehrin E, et al: Quantitative analysis of D2-dopamine receptor binding in the living human brain by PET. Science 231:258–261, 1986

Farde L, Wiesel F-A, Hall H, et al: No D2-receptor increase in PET study of schizophrenia. Arch Gen Psychiatry 44:671–672, 1987

Farde L, Wiesel F-A, Halldin C, et al: Central D2-dopamine receptor occupancy in schizophrenic patients treated with antipsychotic drugs. Arch Gen Psychiatry 45:71–76, 1988

Farde L, Wiesel F-A, Nordström A-L, et al: D1- and D2-dopamine receptor occupancy during treatment with conventional and atypical neuroleptics. Psychopharmacology (Berl) 99:S28–S31, 1989

Gur RE, Resnick SM, Gur RC: Laterality and frontality of cerebral blood flow and metabolism in schizophrenia: relationship to symptom specificity. Psychiatry Res 27:325–334, 1989

Martinot J-L, Peron-Magnan P, Huret J-D, et al: Striatal D2 dopaminergic receptors assessed with positron emission tomography and ([76]Br)bromospiperone in untreated schizophrenic patients. Am J Psychiatry 147:44–50, 1990

Sedvall G: The current status of PET-scanning with respect to schizophrenia. Neuropsychopharmacology 7:41–54, 1992

Sedvall G, Farde L, Persson A, et al: Imaging of neurotransmitter receptors in the living human brain. Arch Gen Psychiatry 43:995–1005, 1986

Wiesel F-A: Positron emission tomography in psychiatry. Psychiatric Developments 1:19–47, 1989

Wik G, Wiesel F-A, Sjögren I, et al: Effects of sulpiride and chlorpromazine on regional cerebral glucose metabolism in schizophrenic patients as determined by positron emission tomography. Psychopharmacology (Berl) 97:309–318, 1989

Wolkin A, Barouche F, Wolf AP, et al: Dopamine blockade and clinical response: evidence for two biological subgroups of schizophrenia. Am J Psychiatry 146:905–908, 1989

Wong DF, Wagner HN, Tune LE, et al: Positron emission tomography reveals elevated D_2-dopamine receptors in drug-naive schizophrenics. Science 234:1558–1563, 1986

Section IV

Treatment of Schizophrenia

Prologue to Section IV

Treatment of Schizophrenia

———◆———

Throughout most of history, the treatment of schizophrenia has been relatively crude. The Greeks and Arabs used tranquil environments, soothing waters, and even religious ceremonies. In less enlightened societies, psychotic patients have often been isolated or incarcerated because of their disturbing or disruptive behavior.

The development of neuroleptic medications in the 1950s represented a major breakthrough in the treatment of schizophrenia. When these drugs were developed, it was hoped that the symptoms of schizophrenia could be markedly diminished or even eradicated through early and effective treatment of the positive psychotic symptoms, followed by good psychosocial rehabilitative treatments. Unfortunately, that hope proved to be false. Although neuroleptic medications have helped significantly, it is now clear that they do not decrease the long-term morbidity of the disorder. The quality of life for schizophrenic patients has been partially improved, in that the majority are now able to live in the community. On the other hand, many continue to experience some positive symptoms, as marked by repeated relapses, and the majority manifest negative symptoms, which prevent them from being able to have normal social interactions, to work, or to return to school.

During the past few years, several new approaches to the development of antipsychotic medications have been proposed. These approaches offer new hope for the treatment of schizophrenia. This work is summarized in two chapters of this section of the book.

In Chapter 9, Dr. Arvid Carlsson describes the attempt to develop a rational pharmacology for schizophrenia, based on what we know about how drugs work and how the brain works. Dr. Carlsson is internationally recognized and admired for his solid and original work on the pathophysiology of schizophrenia; in the 1950s he proposed the "dopamine hypothesis," which remains the leading explanation for the pathophysiology of schizophrenia. This hypothesis was based on the recognition that neuroleptics exert their therapeutic effect through dopamine blockade. Although the dopamine hypothesis probably represents an oversimplification of the complex pathophysiology of schizophrenia, it remains the primary heuristic for understanding how the illness develops and how drugs can be used to treat it.

Dr. Carlsson also presents qualifications and elaborations of the dopamine hypothesis, which emphasize the importance of interactions between the multiple neurotransmitter systems in the brain (e.g., dopamine and glutamate). He describes how insights about multiple drug interactions and the underlying neurochemistry of schizophrenia can be used to develop more "gentle" drugs, such as partial dopamine receptor agonists.

In Chapter 10, Dr. John M. Kane provides a comprehensive overview of neuroleptic treatment of schizophrenia, including the older "typical" compounds and the newer "atypical" neuroleptics. Dr. Kane has been one of the leaders in exploring new neuroleptics, particularly clozapine. As indicated in this chapter, the new atypical neuroleptics affect a variety of neurotransmitter systems, especially serotonin. The old truism that the ideal neuroleptic would be a potent D_2 receptor blocker has been supplemented by the recognition that other neurotransmitter systems may also have important effects on schizophrenia.

In the final chapter of this section, Dr. Thomas H. McGlashan moves from biology back to the human sphere. Not only does Dr. McGlashan provide an excellent overview of the various treatments available, but he also provides an eloquent indictment of treatment approaches that focus only on the "bottom line." He stresses that there is more to the treatment of schizophrenia than the simple reduction of signs and symptoms. Patients with schizophrenia are entitled to receive treatments that will improve their social adjustment and their capacity to work effectively and to engage in the pursuit of happiness. He reminds us that we should not forget the human heritage of Dorothea Dix, Harry Stack Sullivan, and George Brooks, all of whom stressed that the effort to cure must be accompanied by the capacity to care.

Chapter 9

The Search for the Ideal Medications

Developing a Rational Neuropharmacology

Arvid Carlsson, M.D., Ph.D.

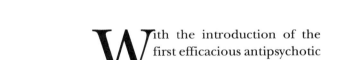

With the introduction of the first efficacious antipsychotic and antidepressant agents in the 1950s, and the subsequent discovery that they act by interfering, in different ways, with neurotransmitter functions in the central nervous system, brain research took a new path. In fact, the discovery of neurohumoral transmission as an important principle in central nervous system function is closely linked to the elucidation of the mode of action of the modern psychopharmacological agents. Moreover, biological psychiatry and neurology have received a tremendous impetus, and neuropsychiatric disorders are now discussed predominantly in terms of neurotransmitter disturbances and imbalances.

Thanks to the powerful tools provided by the modern psychopharmacological agents, it has become possible to approach many neuropsychiatric problems at the molecular level. The focus of interest is in the synapse, with its enzymes involved, for example, in the synthesis and degradation of neurotransmitters, and its transport mechanisms, receptors, secondary and tertiary messengers, and so on. Recently this research area has received a strong impetus from molecular biology. Receptors and other macromolecules engaged in the synaptic transmission can now be investigated with an increasing degree of sophistication.

However, attention must also be devoted to the function of the brain at a higher level of integration. How do the various transmitter systems and neuronal pathways interact? How does the brain function, viewed as a system—the central nervous *system*? A better understanding of the higher integrative functions of the brain will ultimately depend on the further development of this area of research. In fact, the spectacular development at the molecular level has provided research with new, powerful tools to study the higher integrative functions of the brain. Moreover, recent advances in neuroanatomy have paved the way for new strategies to investigate the interaction between different brain regions and neuronal pathways with well-defined neurotransmitter functions (see, e.g., Heimer et al. 1985; Nauta 1989).

The purpose of this chapter is to illustrate how various aspects of modern brain research can lead to new pharmacological concepts and therapeutic principles. Examples are taken from neurotransmission mechanisms in the basal ganglia, including their limbic portions. After discussing new aspects of the pharmacological manipulation of dopaminergic transmission, I widen the perspective in an attempt to open up new possibilities of understanding how dopamine interacts with other important neurotransmitter systems, and how the pharmacological manipulation of these systems may lead to new therapeutic principles.

Shortcomings of the Present Dopaminergic Drugs

Powerful tools are available to manipulate dopaminergic function experimentally as well as therapeutically, in the sense of either stimulation or inhibition. One major problem with dopaminergic stimulants and inhibitors alike is that they tend to exert too drastic acute effects. Moreover, they tend to induce serious perturbations of dopamine function during chronic treatment. Possibly these two phenomena are interrelated. They may both be due to a too brutal treatment of receptors, with deleterious consequences primarily for the receptors themselves, but perhaps secondarily for other neurotransmitter systems in close cooperation with dopamine.

Dopaminergic agonists may easily cause overstimulation, as manifested by involuntary movements, delirious and psychotic states, and emesis. Following chronic treatment of Parkinson's disease, the therapeutic response tends to become less satisfactory, apparently owing to oscillations between over- and understimulation of dopaminergic receptors (the so-called on-off phenomenon). Dopaminergic antagonists, on the other hand, tend to cause serious movement disturbances, which present acutely as parkinsonism, dystonias, akathisia, and related conditions, and chronically as tardive dyskinesias.

It is interesting to note that long-term treatment with antidepressant agents tends to be less problematic than treatment with antipsychotic and antiparkinsonian drugs, at least with respect to the central nervous system. A possible explanation could be that the antidepressants are indirectly acting monoaminergic agonists, whereas the antipsychotic and antiparkinsonian drugs act directly on the receptors. Indirect actions are to a much greater extent under control, for example by feedback mechanisms, thereby preventing excessive changes in receptor activities. One might then be tempted to conclude that future drug development should aim at indirectly acting agonists and antagonists. However, the directly acting receptor ligands have one potentially great advantage: the existence of receptor subtypes offers the opportunity to develop directly acting ligands with selective action on only one subtype, which may improve the balance between therapeutic efficacy and side effects.

If the hypothesis that some important complications of treatment with directly acting receptor ligands are due to too drastic perturbations of receptor function is valid, ways to circumvent this problem must be found. Two alternative strategies will be discussed in the next two sections of this chapter.

Partial Dopamine Receptor Agonists

The use of partial receptor agonists reflects a current trend in drug development away from the earlier effort to develop agonists and antagonists with the highest possible potency and efficacy. The present trend is to develop more "gentle" agents, exemplified by the partial agonists.

A partial receptor agonist is unable to bring about a maximal conformational change of the receptor molecule. This leads to a less-than-maximal so-called intrinsic efficacy. The functional outcome depends on a number of factors. First of all, the responsiveness of the whole receptor complex plays a role. A high responsiveness will show up as a large proportion of "spare receptors," which are redundant in the sense that the response to a "full" agonist will be the same, regardless of their presence or absence. A partial receptor agonist, even though it is unable to bring about a maximal conformational change of the individual receptor molecule, may still be able to stimulate a sufficient number of receptors to induce a full functional response, provided that a sufficient number of spare receptors are present. The partial agonist is then said to have a full intrinsic *activity*, despite having only a partial intrinsic *efficacy*.

Thus, depending on the intrinsic efficacy and the responsiveness of the receptor complex, the degree of stimulation induced by a partial receptor agonist may be higher, equal to, or lower than the receptor stimulation that at a given time is brought about by the endogenous agonist. As a consequence, the partial agonist will appear as an agonist, as an apparently inactive compound, or as an antagonist. A partial receptor agonist is thus also called a mixed agonist/antagonist. Since the responsiveness of the receptor complex varies with the location and with the prevailing physiological conditions, a partial receptor agonist may at any given time present with a mosaic profile of agonistic and antagonistic actions.

Dopaminergic autoreceptors are located primarily outside the synaptic cleft and are thus geared to lower concentrations of the endogenous agonist dopamine than the postsynaptic receptors. As a consequence, partial dopamine receptor agonists generally have a stronger agonistic influence on the autoreceptors than on the postsynaptic receptors. Whether these two receptor types are different subtypes in the sense of being structurally distinct, or they simply represent different conformation states or differ in number of spare receptors, cannot be stated at present. In cases where one aims to utilize the antidopaminergic properties of these agents, as in the treatment of psychoses, an agonistic action on the autoreceptors is favorable, because it contributes to the dampening of dopaminergic activity (for further explanation, see the next section).

Obviously, partial receptor agonists are a challenge to the medicinal chemist. For example, in the treatment of psychotic conditions, one could make use of the fact that in general it takes a lower degree of dopamine receptor blockade to cause an antipsychotic response than to induce extrapyramidal side effects (for a recent, elegant demonstration of this phenomenon using positron-emission tomography [PET], see Farde et al. 1988). Thus it should be theoretically possible to develop a drug with an intrinsic efficacy precisely adequate to allow for a receptor blockade needed for a therapeutic response, yet insufficient to induce extrapyramidal side effects. One might argue that the same goal could be reached simply by carefully controlling the concentration of a classical neuroleptic agent. In principle this is true, but in practice it is rarely possible because of the narrow therapeutic index and the difficulties in keeping drug concentrations constant in body fluids and tissues.

The prototype of partial dopaminergic receptor agonists is the levorotatory form of N-n-propyl-3-(3-hydroxyphenyl)-piperidine (3-PPP) (see Figure 9–1). This agent has been extensively investigated in experimental animals and has been found to possess properties predictive of an antipsychotic action, whereas effects indicative of extrapyramidal side effects are absent (see Clark et al. 1985a, 1985b). It is now in clinical trial. Several other partial dopaminergic receptor agonists with varying intrinsic efficacies are now also in clinical trials. It is hoped that within a few years we will learn whether this principle can be utilized, for example, in the treatment of psychosis, mania, and confusional states.

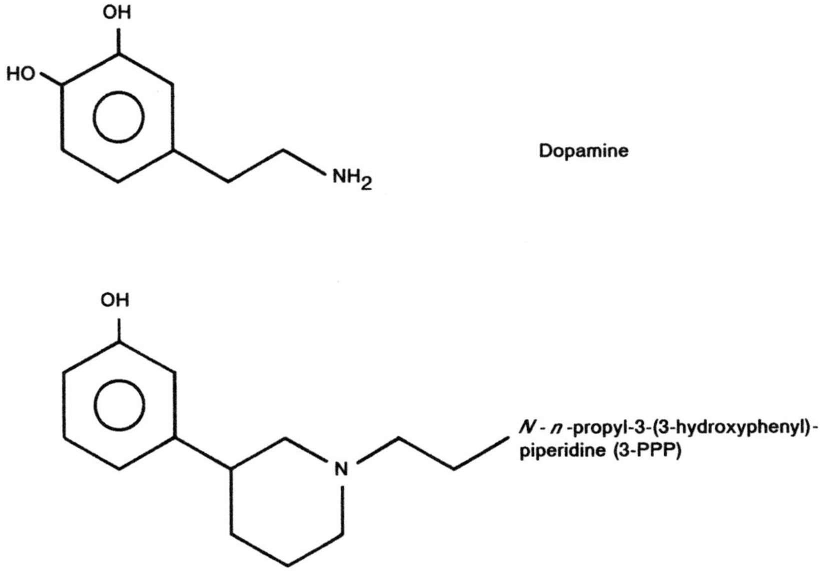

Figure 9–1. Structural formulas of dopamine and N-n-propyl-3-(3-hydroxyphenyl)-piperidine (3-PPP).

Preferential Dopaminergic Autoreceptor Antagonists

An alternative way to manipulate dopaminergic mechanisms in a "gentle," submaximal way is to develop preferential autoreceptor antagonists. Autoreceptors are located on neurons, which produce and release the neurotransmitter to which the autoreceptor is sensitive. When autoreceptors are stimulated by an appropriate agonist, they inhibit the activities of the neuron: autoreceptors located on the soma and dendrites inhibit the firing and those located on the nerve terminals inhibit the release and synthesis of the neurotransmitter. It thus apparently serves as a primitive feedback mechanism.

Whereas the partial dopaminergic agonists previously discussed can show up as agonists or weak antagonists on dopaminergic autoreceptors, leading to inhibition or weak stimulation of dopaminergic neurons, the dopaminergic autoreceptor antagonists always have a stimulating influence on these neurons. Thus they stimulate the firing of the neuron as well as the synthesis and release of the neurotransmitter. The major classical antipsychotic agents act by blocking dopamine receptors postsynaptically, but in addition they block the dopaminergic autoreceptors. This will serve to partially counteract the postsynaptic effect, which, however, will ultimately prevail. Classical antipsychotic agents appear to show a certain preference for blocking autoreceptors, as indicated by slightly stimulating properties in low dosage. However, such an effect usually shows up only within a narrow dose range.

It has been suggested that the antidepressant actions of neuroleptics are due to such preferential action on dopaminergic autoreceptors (see A. Carlsson 1988 [with commentaries and the author's reply]). Preferential autoreceptor antagonists are able to block the autoreceptors at dosage levels that are relatively ineffective in blocking the postsynaptic receptors. As a consequence, preferential dopamine autoreceptor antagonists can act as stronger stimulants and are active over a much wider dose range than the classical neuroleptics. On the other hand, in contrast to classical stimulants such as amphetamine, they are mild stimulants, with a ceiling caused by postsynaptic receptor blockade induced when the dosage is increased. Compounds belonging to this class of agents are (+)-AJ76 and (+)-UH232 (see Svensson et al. 1986a, 1986b; for formulas, see Figure 9–2). The former agent shows a somewhat higher preference for the autoreceptor than the latter.

An interesting feature of the preferential dopamine autoreceptor antagonists is that their activity appears to depend on the baseline activity of the animal. For example, as shown in Figure 9–3, in rats habituated to their environment and thus rather inactive, (+)-UH232 causes a fairly marked increase in locomotor activity, whereas in animals actively exploring a new environment, only a moderate increase in activity is observed; in rats at a very high level of activity induced by a dopaminergic receptor agonist, (+)-UH232 inhibits locomotor activity when given in a dose that causes an increased activity in habituated rats. These data suggest that the balance between the blocking actions on autoreceptors and on postsynaptic receptors, or at least the functional consequences of such actions, depends on the baseline activity of the animal. These agents thus appear to have a stabilizing or normalizing action somewhat reminiscent of lithium. The potential utility of an agent with such properties in various mental disorders seems obvious, not least in schizophrenia, where both positive and negative symptoms may be expected to improve. It is hoped that agents with this profile will be taken to human investigation in the not-too-distant future.

Pharmacological Manipulation of Nervous Pathways Interacting With the Dopaminergic System

Recent observations have disclosed that dopamine does not play as decisive a role in the regulation of psychomotor activity as was formerly

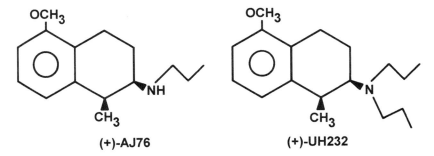

Figure 9–2. Structural formulas for preferential dopamine autoreceptor antagonists. (+)-AJ76 is the *N*-monopropyl and (+)-UH232 the *N,N*-dipropyl derivative.

believed. Thus, even in the virtually complete absence of dopamine in the brain, which leads to almost complete immobility of experimental animals, motility can be induced by manipulating nondopaminergic mechanisms. Drugs acting as antagonists on *N*-methyl-D-aspartic acid (NMDA) receptors (one of the major subtypes of glutamatergic/aspartergic receptors), such as MK-801 or AP-5, are capable of inducing motility under such conditions (M. Carlsson and Carlsson 1989c; M. Carlsson and Svensson 1990).

These observations indicate that a glutamatergic/aspartergic mechanism exerts a powerful inhibitory influence. A reasonable candidate for such activity is the corticostriatal pathway (A. Carlsson 1988) (see Figure 9–4). The striatal complexes appear to serve a powerful inhibitory function on their major targets, the thalamus and the mesencephalic reticular formation, and this inhibition is reinforced by the corticostriatal pathway.

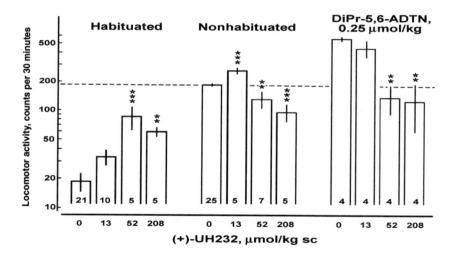

Figure 9–3. Effect of (+)-UH232 on locomotor activity of rats at three different baseline activity levels. *Left:* The rats were habituated to the motility cages for 90 minutes before the measurements of locomotor activity. The drug was injected 35 minutes before the recordings for 30 minutes. *Center:* The drug was injected 5 minutes before the recordings for 30 minutes. *Right:* Racemic 5,6-dihydroxy-2-(di-*n*-propylamino)tetralin HCl, a dopamine-receptor agonist, was injected 60 minutes and (+)-UH232 5 minutes before the activity recordings. Control subjects received saline injections throughout the experiments. [**]$P < .01$; [***]$P < .001$, versus appropriate control. Data compiled from Svensson et al. (1986a, 1986b).

As a consequence of this inhibition I have proposed that the sensory information relayed in the thalamus is largely prevented from reaching the cortex (A. Carlsson 1988). Likewise, the arousal induced by stimuli from the outer world and from the various parts of the body is dampened. The mesostriatal dopamine pathways exert an inhibitory influence on the striatum and thus allow for more information to reach the cortex and to induce arousal. If the flow of information reaching the cerebral cortex is allowed to become excessive, the integrative capacity of the cortex breaks down, and psychosis or delirium may arise.

Phencyclidine (PCP, or angel dust) is an NMDA-receptor antagonist acting on the same site as MK-801. PCP has been found to be capable of inducing disease states mimicking schizophrenia perhaps even more

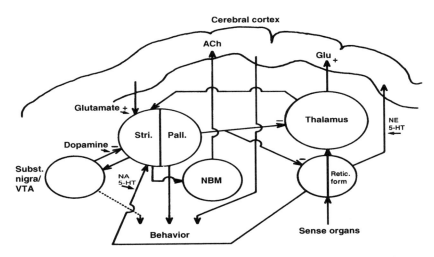

Figure 9–4. Schematic representation of the hypothesis that the cerebral cortex can protect itself from an overload of information and from hyperarousal by means of feedback loops engaging the striatal complexes (Stri./Pall.) and the thalamus/mesencephalic reticular formation (Retic. form.). The striatal complexes, which encompass the dorsal as well as the ventral ("limbic") striatum, are controlled by the cerebral cortex via a glutamatergic/aspartergic excitatory pathway. The mesostriatal dopaminergic inhibitory pathway (from the substantia nigra/ventral tegmental area [Subst. nigra/VTA]) serves to counterbalance the corticostriatal pathway. The influence of the striatal complexes on the thalamus/mesencephalic reticular formation is inhibitory and serves to reduce the sensory input/arousal to the cortex. ACh = acetylcholine. Glu = glutamate. 5-HT = 5-hydroxytryptamine (serotonin). NBM = nucleus basalis of Meynert. NE = norepinephrine.

faithfully than amphetamine. Also, MK-801 appears to be psychotogenic. PCP also has affinity for so-called sigma sites, but this appears to be less important for its pharmacological profile.

From these observations and interpretations it may be inferred that the glutamatergic/aspartergic corticostriatal pathway can be involved in the pathogenesis of schizophrenia and other psychotic conditions, as well as in mania and various confusional states. The development of an NMDA-receptor agonist with satisfactory selectivity for the functions being discussed here might turn out to have considerable clinical utility. Antagonists, on the other hand, might find use in Parkinson's disease, provided that psychotogenic activity can be avoided.

A dramatic potentiation of the motility-inducing action of MK-801 by the α_2-receptor agonist clonidine has been discovered. This effect was found to be resistant against classical neuroleptics, but could be blocked by the "atypical" neuroleptic agent clozapine. The remarkable efficacy and profile of clozapine, with few extrapyramidal side effects, thus may be explained in part by its well-established antiadrenergic action, which may be assumed to potentiate its dopamine-receptor blocking action (M. Carlsson and Carlsson 1989a).

Another remarkable recent observation is the ability of clonidine in combination with atropine to induce motility in dopamine-depleted mice. The motility thus induced differs from that evoked by MK-801. Whereas the motility evoked by MK-801 is clearly abnormal, allowing almost exclusively for forward locomotion in the mouse, the motility induced by clonidine plus atropine looks like normal exploratory activity. These observations suggest that the influence of the glutamatergic/aspartergic system on psychomotor activity is selective and may serve to initiate behavioral programs adequate for the actual situation. Perhaps this function is mainly exerted by inhibiting less purposeful behavioral programs (see M. Carlsson and Carlsson 1989b).

These observations draw attention to both adrenergic and cholinergic mechanisms. Perhaps the potential of manipulating these mechanisms in the treatment of psychiatric disorders, including schizophrenia, should be revisited in light of recent evidence.

References

Carlsson A: The current status of the dopamine hypothesis of schizophrenia. Neuropsychopharmacology 1:179–186, 1988

Carlsson M, Carlsson A: Dramatic synergism between MK-801 and clonidine with respect to locomotor stimulatory effect in monoamine-depleted mice. Journal of Neural Transmission 77:65–71, 1989a

Carlsson M, Carlsson A: Marked locomotor stimulation in monoamine-depleted mice following treatment with atropine in combination with clonidine. J Neural Transm Park Dis Dement Sect 1:317–322, 1989b

Carlsson M, Carlsson A: The NMDA antagonist MK-801 causes marked locomotor stimulation in monoamine-depleted mice. Journal of Neural Transmission 75:221–226, 1989c

Carlsson M, Svensson A: Interfering with glutamatergic neurotransmission by means of MK-801 administration discloses the locomotor stimulatory potential of other transmitter systems in rats and mice. Pharmacol Biochem Behav 36:45–50, 1990

Clark D, Hjorth S, Carlsson A: Dopamine receptor agonists: mechanisms underlying autoreceptor selectivity, I: review of the evidence. Journal of Neural Transmission 62:1–52, 1985a

Clark D, Hjorth S, Carlsson A: Dopamine receptor agonists: mechanisms underlying autoreceptor selectivity, II: theoretical considerations. Journal of Neural Transmission 62:171–207, 1985b

Farde L, Wiesel F-A, Halldin C, et al: Central D_2-dopamine receptor occupancy in schizophrenic patients treated with antipsychotic drugs. Arch Gen Psychiatry 45:71–76, 1988

Heimer L, Alheid GF, Zaborszky L: Basal ganglia, in The Rat Nervous System, Vol 1: Forebrain and Midbrain. Edited by Paxinos G. New York, Academic Press, 1985, pp 37–86

Nauta WJF: Reciprocal links of the corpus striatum with the cerebral cortex and limbic system: a common substrate for movement and thought, in Neurology and Psychiatry: A Meeting of Minds. Edited by Mueller J. Basel, Karger, 1989, pp 43–63

Svensson K, Johansson AM, Magnusson T, et al: (+)-AJ76 and (+)-UH232: central stimulants acting as preferential dopamine autoreceptor antagonists. Naunyn Schmiedeberg's Arch Pharmacol 334:234–245, 1986a

Svensson K, Hjorth S, Clark D, et al: (+)-UH232 and (+)-UH242: novel stereoselective DA receptor antagonists with preferential action on autoreceptors. Journal of Neural Transmission 65:1–27, 1986

Chapter 10

Efficacy, Mechanisms, and Side Effects of Typical and Atypical Neuroleptics

John M. Kane, M.D.

T he clinical therapeutic and adverse effects of neuroleptic drugs have provided both impetus and direction for exploring potential mechanisms of action for these compounds. The introduction of "atypical" antipsychotic medications has added a new dimension to research in this area. In this chapter, I briefly review several areas relevant to further understanding of clinical drug effects and potential mechanisms of action.

Efficacy

The efficacy of neuroleptic medications has been demonstrated in numerous double-blind placebo-controlled trials in acute, continuation, and maintenance treatment of schizophrenia. There are several features of clinical response, however, that need to be taken into consideration in discussing mechanism of action and potential differences between compounds.

Heterogeneity of drug response remains an important phenomenon. Given the presumed heterogeneity of schizophrenia, variations in drug response might be anticipated. It is likely that some clinical trials of neuroleptic medications include placebo responders as well as patients who may be unresponsive to any medication. In exploring mechanisms of action via in vivo changes in specific neurochemicals, neuromodulators, and receptor phenomena, it would be ideal to focus only on those individuals who have a clear therapeutic response to the compound in question.

Dose-response relationships for a given compound and dose equivalency estimates between different compounds become critical in exploring hypotheses regarding mechanisms. Despite years of clinical experience and countless clinical trials, this remains an area with few hard facts. For example, discussions of specific receptor effects postulated as important are based on assumptions regarding effective dosage equivalence between various compounds (Creese et al. 1976; Seeman et al. 1976).

Klein and Davis (1969) reviewed an extensive series of double-blind placebo-controlled studies and found that those trials employing dosages of chlorpromazine in excess of 400 mg/day were consistent in demonstrating superiority of chlorpromazine, but those studies employing a lower dose were by and large unable to demonstrate a significant drug effect. McEvoy et al. (1991) reported that 75% of a sample of schizophrenic or schizoaffective patients responded to a dose of haloperidol averaging 3.7 mg ($\pm$ 2.3 mg) daily. Most dose equivalency tables would equate this to 200 mg/day of chlorpromazine. Interestingly, McEvoy et al. found significantly better response among acute and subacute patients as compared with those who had been continuously psychotic for more than 6 months. (The focus of this investigation on the "neuroleptic threshold" hypothesis is discussed later in this chapter in relation to adverse effects.) There may be differences in terms of dose-response relationships based on stage of illness and prior length and dose of neuroleptic treatment, but systematic studies capable of addressing this question are lacking.

Given enormous individual variability in absorption and metabolism of neuroleptic medications, there have been numerous attempts to assess the relationship between blood levels and clinical response (either therapeutic or adverse effects). It was hoped that this strategy would go a long way toward helping to explain the enormous heterogeneity in drug response seen among patients with schizophrenia. To a large extent these hopes have not been fulfilled, and methodology in this area remains a problem.

The most widely studied drug has been haloperidol, and several investigations with this compound (and some with fluphenazine) have suggested a curvilinear relationship between blood levels and clinical response, or a putative "therapeutic window" (e.g., Garver et al. 1984; Mavroidis et al. 1983, 1984; van Putten et al. 1989). Although these findings are intriguing, more studies are necessary to establish the validity of this hypothesis. Some investigators have failed to find a curvilinear relationship, and some studies have included few patients above the suggested upper limit. More importantly, few attempts have been made to randomly assign patients whose blood levels are out of the therapeutic range to a dosage necessary to manipulate the blood level into the putative therapeutic range or to remain at their current blood level (to control for continued time on drug). Until this is done in a systematic, reproducible fashion, it is difficult to draw meaningful conclusions. Another important issue in evaluating the hypothesis of a therapeutic window is the possibility that some of those patients showing minimal or poor response at higher blood levels may be experiencing behaviorally manifest adverse effects that could alter or impair the therapeutic response (Bolvig-Hansen et al. 1982). This issue is potentially important in that if a curvilinear relationship does exist, then this requires an explanation of the pharmacodynamic or receptor effects that would be consistent with this phenomenon.

The assumed equal efficacy among neuroleptic drugs is another important consideration in exploring mechanisms of action. With the recent exception of clozapine (Kane et al. 1988), there are no convincing data that among medications marketed in the United States, any one is more effective either in schizophrenia in general or in specific subtypes of the disorder. It is certainly possible that differences do exist, but that appropriate studies have not been conducted to identify them. Few studies provide generalizable data on differential treatment response to specific agents. The available data base is derived from comparisons of overall response rate in group data contrasting one drug with another. Even if similar proportions of patients respond to each drug, this does not necessarily mean that a given individual would respond equally well to both drugs. Despite the obvious clinical importance of this issue, remarkably few studies (e.g., Gardos 1978) have addressed this question. Although anecdotal reports suggest that a patient who fails to respond to one drug might occasionally benefit from another drug, it is difficult to establish a cause-and-effect relationship in a single case because other factors—such as additional time on medication—could contribute to improvement.

Time Course of Response

There is considerable heterogeneity in time course of response, and this phenomenon has been a challenge to the investigation of neurochemical mechanisms. Most controlled clinical trials in acutely psychotic patients last a matter of weeks, but the full therapeutic gains derived from antipsychotic medications are not seen for several weeks and in some cases for several months. Dopamine receptor blockade, on the other hand, occurs within hours following neuroleptic administration (see the next section of this chapter).

The length of time that a patient has been ill prior to the initiation of drug therapy may have some influence on treatment response. This raises an interesting question regarding neurochemical mechanisms, although one could hypothesize other factors that might be responsible for this finding. May et al. (1976) conducted a 3- to 5-year follow-up study of first-admission patients who at their index episode had been randomly assigned to antipsychotic drugs, psychotherapy, psychotherapy plus drugs, electroconvulsive therapy, or placebo. Those patients who had not received medication or electroconvulsive therapy during the index episode spent significantly more time in hospital during the follow-up interval, despite the fact that these patients were subsequently treated with medication.

Other investigations have suggested a relationship between length of illness prior to the initiation of drug therapy and treatment outcome (Crow et al. 1986; Rabiner et al. 1986). These studies, however, did not involve random assignment to drug or placebo for the treatment of the index episode, and insidious onset and/or not seeking or accepting treatment for long periods may indicate a poor prognosis.

Most of the focus on clinical implications for mechanism has been on acute response. Attention should also be given to "offset" as well as onset of clinical response. How do we explain the enormous heterogeneity in time course of relapse following neuroleptic withdrawal, and how do we account for those psychotic relapses that occur during maintenance treatment?

The ability of dopamine agonists (e.g., methylphenidate, amphetamine, L-dopa) to produce transient exacerbations of psychosis in remitted patients receiving neuroleptic medication is also a reproducible clinical phenomenon that has implications for neurochemical mechanisms (Angrist et al. 1980, 1985; Lieberman et al. 1984, 1987). The observation by Lieberman et al. (1987) that concomitant neuroleptic treatment has minimal attenuation effect on this phenomenon when response is contrasted in the same patients, both on and off drug, is also intriguing and requires explanation.

Another critical issue in exploring mechanisms is the development of adverse effects, particularly neurologic effects—both acute and chronic. Here, too, heterogeneity is a critical factor; not all patients develop acute extrapyramidal side effects and not all patients develop chronic effects such as tardive dyskinesia or tardive dystonia. In addition, most of the focus on tardive dyskinesia has involved explorations regarding etiology, but heterogeneity in phenomenology, outcome, and treatment response is also critical and may be very informative regarding drug mechanisms. For example, some patients develop a very-rapid-onset and severe form of tardive dyskinesia, whereas others develop mild cases that are not progressive and may even improve over time despite continued neuroleptic administration. In addition, if specific subgroups of patients are more vulnerable (e.g., those with affective disorders), what clues might this provide for exploring mechanisms?

Dopamine Hypothesis

The identification of dopamine and an appreciation of its role as a neurotransmitter, combined with ongoing efforts to map dopaminergic pathways and to establish its role in influencing a variety of behavioral phenomena, have been of enormous importance. Equally important have been the identification of dopamine deficiency in Parkinson's disease and the observations that neuroleptic drugs characteristically act as antagonists at dopamine receptors. It was also very encouraging when investigators were able to demonstrate correlations between the neuroleptic daily dosage necessary for clinical efficacy and neuroleptic affinity for the D_2 receptor (Creese et al. 1976; Seeman 1980; Seeman et al. 1976). More recent reanalysis (Seeman 1992) suggests that clozapine does not fit well in this correlation; however, clozapine's affinity for the D_4 receptor may explain its atypicality in this regard.

As previously mentioned, one apparent difficulty in exploring mechanisms of action is the inability to reconcile the rapid dopamine receptor blockade following administration of neuroleptic drugs and the time course of therapeutic effect, which is both varied and substantially longer than a few days. Bunney and Grace (1978) and Chiodo and Bunney

(1983) utilized extracellular single unit recording techniques to study the effects of both acute and repeated oral neuroleptic administration on the in vivo activity of rat A9 and A10 dopaminergic neurons. These investigators demonstrated significant differences between the effects of short- and long-term drug administration. Short-term administration produced a large increase in spontaneous firing rate, whereas long-term administration produced a reduction in the basal firing rate of the same neurons—a tonic depolarization blockade.

Pickar et al. (1986) reported time-dependent changes in levels of plasma homovanillic acid (HVA) occurring during both neuroleptic treatment and withdrawal and suggested that the neuroleptic-induced, time-dependent decrease observed in plasma HVA and its correlation with clinical response share some similarities with the preclinical model proposed by Bunney (1988). Earlier studies by Bowers and Swigar (1987) had also suggested that those patients sharing a good response to neuroleptics had significantly higher pretreatment HVA levels than did patients with poorer response and that significant decreases in plasma HVA during the first few weeks of neuroleptic treatment were found in those who responded well clinically.

Effects of Typical and Atypical Drugs

A distinct problem remains in the terminology employed to discuss putative neuroleptic drugs. Many authors have used the term "atypical neuroleptic," but a frequently cited distinguishing feature of these drugs is their lack of neuroleptic properties (Kane et al. 1988). There is no consistent, well-validated criteria set to differentiate typical from atypical drugs. In general, the atypical drugs are felt to be more specific for a given type of dopamine receptor, less likely to produce neurologic side effects, and/or less likely to produce elevations in prolactin (Deutch et al. 1991). Clearly, this represents a diverse group of characteristics not necessarily related to each other or derived from some common mechanistic explanation. In addition, it is unclear to what extent these characteristics can be reliably determined prior to their introduction into the clinic.

Clozapine has served as somewhat of a model in developing atypical compounds and has stimulated research to establish putative mechanisms for its novel effects. Early observations in the clinic suggested that clozapine was relatively free of acute extrapyramidal side effects. Subsequently, this compound was shown to be superior to control drugs (haloperidol and chlorpromazine) in the treatment of carefully selected patients with a documented history of poor response to neuroleptic drugs (Kane et al. 1988). In addition, clozapine produces very modest and somewhat transient elevations in prolactin (Kane et al. 1981), and with more long-term experience it is now reasonably safe to say that clozapine shows a markedly reduced or no propensity to produce tardive dyskinesia or tardive dystonia.

In preclinical studies clozapine was found to be virtually free of cataleptogenic activity and to only weakly antagonize apomorphine- or amphetamine-induced stereotypy (Stille and Hippius 1971). In addition, chronic administration of clozapine does not induce dopaminergic supersensitivity (Sayers et al. 1975). In the model (previously described) employed by Chiodo and Bunney (1983), repeated treatment with clozapine resulted in depolarization inactivation of A10 neurons but not A9 cells. Bunney (1988) also reported that if one combines haloperidol with either an anticholinergic drug such as trihexyphenidyl or an α-blocker such as prazosin, and administers the combination repeatedly, the result is a midbrain dopamine cell activity profile identical to that of clozapine (e.g., inactivation of A10 but not A9 neurons).

The mechanism of clozapine's effect in the depolarization blockade model is interesting. Whether clozapine's pronounced cholinergic and α-adrenergic affinity is relevant is far from clear. Combining atropine with haloperidol, for example, does not fully mimic the pharmacologic properties of clozapine. Haloperidol still inhibits apomorphine-induced circling behavior in caudate-lesioned rats when combined with atropine, whereas clozapine does not (Coward et al. 1989). In addition, the chronic administration of anticholinergic agents with typical neuroleptics does not appear to prevent or reduce the incidence of tardive dyskinesia occurring in clinical populations, nor does it prevent the increase in striatal D_2 receptor density produced by typical neuroleptics (Boyson et al. 1988; Carvey et al. 1988).

Interestingly, other data suggest that dopaminergic mechanisms may play an important role in clozapine's effects. Our group (J. M. Kane et al., unpublished data) has found that among 35 treatment-refractory schizophrenic patients treated for 6 weeks with clozapine, the 15 patients who met a priori criteria for response had significantly higher prolactin levels at weeks 3 and 4 than those 20 patients who did not meet criteria for response. This difference was apparent despite the fact that clozapine in general produces very slight and transient elevations in prolactin.

Coward et al. (1989) suggested that, given the possible importance of GABAergic functional involvement in the pathophysiology of tardive dyskinesia (Gunne et al. 1984), clozapine's effects on this system may be particularly relevant. Chronic administration of typical neuroleptics reduces gamma-aminobutyric acid (GABA) turnover within the substantia nigra of the rat, and GABAergic supersensitivity has been described within this region (Coward 1982; Frey et al. 1987; Gale 1980). Coward (1982) showed that, in contrast, nigral GABA sensitivity is slightly reduced after short-term withdrawal from chronic clozapine exposure but is increased after 1 week. This increased sensitivity of nigral GABAergic systems then declines, with no differences being observed between placebo-, haloperidol-, and clozapine-treated rats after 14 days' withdrawal from treatment.

Serotonin

Altar et al. (1983), Schmidt and Seeger (1986), and Meltzer et al. (1989) suggested that many so-called atypical drugs such as clozapine have more potent antiserotonergic (against 5-HT$_2$) than antidopaminergic (against D$_2$) activity, which may contribute to their apparent lower probability of extrapyramidal side effects. These investigators examined a range of antipsychotic agents and reported greater 5-HT$_2$-to-D$_2$ ratios for those drugs with lower probability of extrapyramidal side effects.

Casey (1989), on the other hand, tested 20 cebus monkeys with compounds that ranged from high to very low D$_2$-to-S$_2$ ratios (specifically haloperidol, clopenthixol, tefludazine, and setoperone), but all drugs produced clinically indistinguishable dose-related dystonia with similar dose thresholds. This is in contrast to the previously cited rodent studies (Altar et al. 1983; Meltzer et al. 1989; Schmidt and Seeger 1986).

Clozapine's effects on serotonergic systems have been studied indirectly in the clinic. Clozapine was shown to inhibit the cortisol response to MK-212, a directly acting 5-HT agonist (Lowy et al. 1988). This effect of MK-212 on cortisol was not inhibited by chlorpromazine, molindone, or haloperidol (Meltzer et al. 1989), despite the fact that chlorpromazine has an affinity similar to that of clozapine for the 5-HT$_2$ receptor in vitro. The implications of this finding remain to be determined; perhaps clozapine is more potent in vivo or the 5-HT$_2$ receptor is not the only system involved in MK-212's effects.

Lemus et al. (1991) conducted a fenfluramine challenge test in seven treatment-refractory schizophrenic patients before and after short-term (2 to 3 weeks) clozapine treatment. Clozapine significantly inhibited the prolactin response to fenfluramine, suggesting that clozapine affects serotonin receptors at least in this system.

There are a variety of suggested interactions between the serotonergic and dopaminergic systems in various brain regions. The extent to which abnormalities in serotonergic systems in patients with schizophrenia are implied by these findings is unclear.

There have been some reports of diminished 5-HT_2 receptors in postmortem tissue from midfrontal gyrus and anterior cingulate gyrus of schizophrenic patients as compared with control subjects (Laruelle et al. 1990), but these patients had received neuroleptics, which may have produced downregulation of 5-HT_2 receptors. If 5-HT_2 receptors are reduced in schizophrenia independent of the neuroleptic effect, then we need to explain the effects of 5-HT_2 antagonists, which might be expected to worsen the condition.

An interesting pilot study was conducted by Louwerens et al. (1990), who added ritanserin to typical neuroleptics in refractory patients and found no increase in therapeutic effect against positive or negative symptoms. Then the patients were switched to clozapine and showed improvement. Clearly this is not an adequate test of this hypothesis, but few clinical data are available that are truly relevant.

Several compounds (e.g., risperidone) with high 5-HT_2-to-D_2 ratios are now available; also available are compounds that may be relatively specific antagonists at 5-HT_2 or 5-HT_3 receptors. As a result, considerable new information on the importance of serotonin receptor effects should be forthcoming.

Norepinephrine

Considerable research has implicated abnormalities in norepinephrine as playing a potential role in the pathophysiology of schizophrenia and the response to pharmacologic agents (Hornykiewicz 1982; van Kammen and Gelernter 1987). Stein and Wise (1971) proposed that negative symptoms such as anhedonia and loss of drive in schizophrenia were due to a deterioration in central noradrenergic pathways mediating reward response, as evidenced by a decrease in the norepinephrine-synthesizing enzyme dopamine β-hydroxylase. It was reported by van Kammen et al. (1990) that drug-free cerebrospinal fluid (CSF) norepinephrine and 3-methoxy-4-hydroxyphenylglycol levels correlated significantly with the severity of negative symptom and psychosis ratings. Other investigators (Hornykiewicz 1982; van Kammen and Antelman 1984) also found CSF norepinephrine to be increased in schizophrenic patients.

In addition, there has been some suggestion that propranolol, a β-adrenergic receptor blocker, may have therapeutic potential in schizophrenia (Donaldson et al. 1986).

Clozapine has considerable potency as an α-adrenergic antagonist. Clozapine has been shown to increase levels of CSF norepinephrine (Lieberman et al. 1991) to a greater extent than other neurotransmitters studied. There are a variety of ways in which dopamine and norepinephrine may influence each other (e.g., Glowinski et al. 1988), and one can only speculate as to what role this particular property of clozapine might have in its overall efficacy or in its apparent superiority for the reduction of negative symptoms (in treatment-refractory patients who also have positive symptoms).

D_1 Receptor Effects

The role of D_1 receptors in the effects of typical and atypical neuroleptics remains unclear. Although considerable time has elapsed since the initial evidence that dopamine receptors could be subclassified, it has only been in the past 5 years that the first selective D_1 antagonists were available for preclinical studies, and clinical studies are currently under way. In some preclinical studies, D_1 antagonists reproduce many of the functional effects of typical neuroleptics and of selective D_2 antagonists. In addition, these compounds are active in many of the animal and behavioral models predictive of antipsychotic efficacy (Murray and Waddington 1990; Waddington 1989). There is also increasing evidence that D_1 and D_2 receptor stimulation or antagonism may have a variety of interactions or synergistic effects in affecting dopamine-mediated behavioral phenomena.

Farde et al. (1989, 1990), using positron-emission tomography and the selective ligands ^{11}C-SCH 23390 and ^{11}C-raclopride examined central D_1 and D_2 receptor occupancy in schizophrenic patients treated with clinical doses of classical and atypical neuroleptics. Interestingly, of those compounds studied, clozapine appeared to produce the lowest D_2 receptor occupancy and the highest D_1 receptor occupancy. These authors suggested that the mechanism underlying the atypical properties of clozapine may be related to an effect on both D_1 and D_2 receptors. The importance of D_1 receptors will be clarified only by controlled clinical trials with selective D_1 antagonists and by studies of other drugs with D_1/D_2 profiles similar to those of clozapine, but this may prove to be an important line of investigation.

The recent identification, cloning, and sequencing of D_3, D_4, and D_5 receptors raise new possibilities regarding novel mechanisms (Seeman 1990; Sokoloff et al. 1990; Sunahara et al. 1991; Van Tol et al. 1991), which will be actively explored in the near future.

Conclusion

Clearly, enormous progress has been made in studying a variety of receptor systems and receptor subtypes. An increasing array of compounds are now available for preclinical and clinical studies in this research area. These compounds may prove to be useful tools for elucidating those receptor effects responsible for various clinical phenomena, both therapeutic and adverse. At present there is reason to pursue a variety of interesting leads, but there are insufficient data on which to draw meaningful conclusions regarding what is responsible for the apparent novel effects of particular antipsychotic compounds such as clozapine.

References

Altar CA, Wasley DM, Neale RF, et al: Typical and atypical antipsychotic occupancy of D_2 and S_2 receptors: an autoradiographic study in rat brain. Brain Res Bull 16:517–525, 1983

Angrist B, Rosen J, Gershein SL: Responses to apomorphine, amphetamine and neuroleptics in schizophrenic subjects. Psychopharmacology (Berl) 67:31–38, 1980

Angrist B, Peselow E, Rubinstein M, et al: Amphetamine response and relapse risk after depot neuroleptic discontinuation. Psychopharmacology (Berl) 85:277–283, 1985

Bolvig-Hansen LB, Larsen NE, Gulmann N: Dose response relationship of perphenazine in the treatment of acute psychosis. Psychopharmacology (Berl) 78:112–115, 1982

Bowers MB, Swigar ME: Acute psychosis and plasma catecholamine metabolites (letter). Arch Gen Psychiatry 44:190, 1987

Boyson SJ, McGonigle P, Luthin GR, et al: Effects of chronic administration of neuroleptic and anticholinergic agents on the densities of D-2 dopamine and muscarinic cholinergic receptors in rat striatum. J Pharmacol Exp Ther 244:987–993, 1988

Bunney BS: Effects of acute and chronic neuroleptic treatment on the activity of midbrain dopamine neurons. Ann NY Acad Sci 537:77–85, 1988

Bunney BS, Grace AA: Acute and chronic haloperidol treatment: comparison of effects on nigral dopaminergic activity. Life Sci 23:1715–1728, 1978

Carvey PM, Hitri A, Goetz CG, et al: Concurrent treatment with benztropine and haloperidol attenuates development of behavioral hypersensitivity but not dopamine receptor proliferation. Life Sci 42:2207–2215, 1988

Casey DE: Serotonergic aspects of acute extrapyramidal syndromes in nonhuman primates. Psychopharmacol Bull 25:457–459, 1989

Chiodo LA, Bunney BS: Typical and atypical neuroleptics: differential effects of chronic administration on the activity of A9 and A10 midbrain dopaminergic neurons. J Neurosci 3:1607–1619, 1983

Coward DM: Classical and non-classical neuroleptics induce supersensitivity of nigral GABA-ergic mechanisms in the rat. Psychopharmacology (Berl) 78:180–184, 1982

Coward DM, Imperato A, Urwyler S, et al: Biochemical and behavioral properties of clozapine. Psychopharmacology (Berl) 99:S6–S12, 1989

Creese I, Burt DR, Snyder SH: Dopamine receptor binding predicts clinical and pharmacological potencies of antischizophrenic drugs. Science 192:481–483, 1976

Crow TJ, McMillan JF, Johnson AL, et al: The Northwick Park study of first episodes of schizophrenia, II: a randomized controlled trial of prophylactic neuroleptic treatments. Br J Psychiatry 148:120–127, 1986

Deutch AY, Moghaddam B, Innis RB, et al: Mechanisms of action of atypical antipsychotic drugs: implications for novel therapeutic strategies for schizophrenia. Schizophr Res 4:121–156, 1991

Donaldson SR, Gelenberg AJ, Baldessarini RJ: Alternative treatments for schizophrenic psychoses, in American Handbook of Psychiatry. Edited by Arieti. New York, Basic Books, 1986

Farde L, Wiesel S-A, Nordstrom A-L, et al: D-1 and D-2 dopamine receptor occupancy during treatment with conventional and atypical neuroleptics. Psychopharmacology (Berl) 99:S28–S31, 1989

Farde L, Nordstrom A-L, Wiesel F-A, et al: D-1 and D-2 dopamine receptor occupancy during treatment with classical and atypical neuroleptics. Paper presented at the 5th Biennial Winter Workshop on Schizophrenia, Badgastein, Austria, January 28–February 3, 1990

Frey JM, Ticku MK, Huffman RD: GABAergic supersensitivity within the pars reticulata of the rat substantia nigra following chronic haloperidol administration. Brain Res 425:73–84, 1987

Gale K: Chronic blockade of dopamine receptors by antischizophrenic drugs enhances GABA binding in substantia nigra. Nature 283:569–570, 1980

Gardos G: Are antipsychotic drugs interchangeable? J Nerv Ment Dis 159:343–348, 1978

Garver DL, Hirschowitz J, Glickstein GA, et al: Haloperidol, plasma and red blood cell levels in clinical antipsychotic response. J Clin Psychopharmacol 4:133–137, 1984

Glowinski J, Herve D, Tassin JP: Heterologous regulation of receptors on target cells of dopamine neurons in the pre-frontal cortex, nucleus accumbens, and striatum. Ann N Y Acad Sci 537:112–123, 1988

Gunne L-M, Haggstrom J-E, Sjoquist B: Association with persistent neuroleptic-induced dyskinesia of regional changes in brain GABA synthesis. Nature 309:347–349, 1984

Hornykiewicz O: Brain catecholamines in schizophrenia: a good case for noradrenaline. Nature 299:484–486, 1982

Kane JM, Cooper TB, Sachar EJ, et al: Clozapine: plasma levels and prolactin response. Psychopharmacology (Berl) 73:184–187, 1981

Kane J, Honigfeld G, Singer J, et al: Clozapine for the treatment resistant schizophrenic: a double-blind comparison versus chlorpromazine/benztropine. Arch Gen Psychiatry 45:789–796, 1988

Klein DF, Davis JM: Drug Treatment of Psychiatric Disorders. Baltimore, MD, Williams & Wilkins, 1969

Laruelle M, Casanova M, Weinberger DR, et al: Post-mortem study of the dopaminergic D-1 receptors in the dorsolateral prefrontal cortex of schizophrenics and controls. Presented at the 5th Biennial Winter Workshop on Schizophrenia, Badgastein, Austria, January 28–February 3, 1990

Lemus CZ, Lieberman JA, Johns CA, et al: Hormonal responses to fenfluramine challenges in clozapine-treated schizophrenic patients. Biol Psychiatry 29:691–694, 1991

Lieberman JA, Kane JM, Gadaletta D, et al: Methylphenidate challenge as a predictor of relapse in schizophrenia. Am J Psychiatry 141:633–638, 1984

Lieberman J, Kane JM, Sarantakos S, et al: Prediction of relapse in schizophrenia. Arch Gen Psychiatry 44:597–603, 1987

Lieberman J, Johns C, Pollack S, et al: Biochemical effects of clozapine in cerebrospinal fluid of patients with schizophrenia, in Schizophrenia Research: Advances in Neuropsychiatry and Psychopharmacology, Vol 1. Edited by Schulz SC, Tamminga CA. New York, Raven, 1991, pp 341–349

Louwerens JW, Coppens HC, Korf J, et al: On the pathogenetic role of dopaminergic and serotonergic neurotransmission in long-term hospitalized psychotic patients. Presented at the 5th Biennial Winter Workshop on Schizophrenia, Badgastein, Austria, January 28–February 3, 1990

Lowy MT, Koenig JI, Meltzer HY: Stimulation of serum cortisol and prolactin in man by MK-212, a centrally active serotonin agonist. Biol Psychiatry 23:818–828, 1988

Mavroidis ML, Kantor DR, Hirschowitz J, et al: Clinical response and plasma haloperidol levels in schizophrenia. Psychopharmacology (Berl) 81:354–356, 1983

Mavroidis ML, Kantor DR, Hirschowitz J, et al: Therapeutic blood levels of fluphenazine: plasma or RBC determinations? Psychopharmacol Bull 20:168–170, 1984

May PRA, Tuma AH, Yale C, et al: Schizophrenia—a follow-up study of results of treatment, II: hospital stay over 2–5 years. Arch Gen Psychiatry 33:481–486, 1976

McEvoy JP, Hogarty GE, Steingard S: Optimal dose of neuroleptic in acute schizophrenia: a controlled study of the neuroleptic threshold and higher haloperidol dose. Arch Gen Psychiatry 48:739–745, 1991

Meltzer HY, Bastani B, Ramirez L, et al: Clozapine: new research on efficacy and mechanism of action. European Archives of Psychiatry and Neurological Sciences 238:332–339, 1989

Murray AM, Waddington JL: The interaction of clozapine with dopamine D_1 versus dopamine D_2 receptor–mediated function: behavioral indices. Eur J Pharmacol 186:79–86, 1990

Pickar D, Labarca R, Duran AR, et al: Longitudinal measurement of plasma homovanillic acid in schizophrenic patients: correlation with psychosis and response to neuroleptic treatment. Arch Gen Psychiatry 43:669–676, 1986

Rabiner CJ, Wegner JT, Kane JM: Outcome study of first-episode psychosis, I: relapse rates after one year. Am J Psychiatry 143:1155–1158, 1986

Sayers A, Burki H, Ruch W, et al: Neuroleptic-induced hyposensitivity of striatal dopamine receptors in the rat as a model of tardive dyskinesia: effects of clozapine, haloperidol, loxapine and chlorpromazine. Psychopharmacologia 41:97–104, 1975

Schmidt AW, Seeger TF: Serotonin 5-HT-2 potency as a predictor of antipsychotic side effect liability. Society for Neuroscience Abstracts 12:479, 1986

Seeman P: Brain dopamine receptors. Pharmacol Rev 32:229–313, 1980

Seeman P: Atypical neuroleptics: role of multiple receptors, endogenous dopamine, and receptor linkage. Acta Psychiatr Scand Suppl 359:14–20, 1990

Seeman P: Dopamine receptor sequences: therapeutic levels of neuroleptics occupy D_2 receptors, clozapine occupies D_4. Neuropsychopharmacology 7:261–284, 1992

Seeman P, Lee T, Chau-Wong M, et al: Antipsychotic drug doses and neuroleptic/dopamine receptors. Nature 261:717–719, 1976

Sokoloff P, Giros B, Martres MP, et al: Molecular cloning and characterization of a novel dopamine receptor (D_3) as a target for neuroleptics. Nature 347:146–151, 1990

Stein L, Wise CD: Possible etiology of schizophrenia: progressive damage to the noradrenergic reward system by 5-hydroxydopamine. Science 171:1032–1036, 1971

Stille G, Hippius H: Kritische Stellungsnahme zum Begriff der Neuroleptika (anhand von pharmakologischen und klinischen Befunden mit Clozapin). Pharmacopsychiatry 4:182–191, 1971

Sunahara RK, Guan H-C, O'Dowd BF, et al: Cloning of the gene for a human D_5 receptor with higher affinity for dopamine than D_1. Nature 350:614–616, 1991

van Kammen DP, Antelman SM: Impaired noradrenergic transmission in schizophrenia? a mini review. Life Sci 34:1403–1413, 1984

van Kammen DP, Gelernter J: Biochemical instability in schizophrenia, I: the norepinephrine system. In Psychopharmacology, The Third Generation of Progress. Edited by Meltzer HY. New York, Raven, 1987, pp 745–752

van Kammen DP, Peters J, Yao J, et al: Norepinephrine in acute exacerbations of chronic schizophrenia. Arch Gen Psychiatry 47:161–168, 1990

van Putten T, Marder SR, Mintz J, et al: Haloperidol plasma levels and clinical response: a therapeutic window relationship. In Schizophrenia: Scientific Progress. Edited by Schulz SC, Tamminga C. New York, Oxford University Press, 1989, pp 325–332

Van Tol HHM, Bunzow JR, Guan H-C, et al: Cloning of the gene for a human dopamine D_4 receptor with high affinity for the antipsychotic clozapine. Nature 350:610–614, 1991

Waddington JL: Implications of recent research on dopamine D-1 and D-2 receptor subtypes in relation to schizophrenia and neuroleptic drug action. Current Opinion in Psychiatry 2:89–92, 1989

Chapter 11

Psychosocial Treatments of Schizophrenia

The Potential of Relationships

Thomas H. McGlashan, M.D.

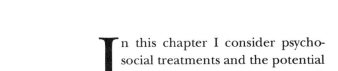

In this chapter I consider psychosocial treatments and the potential of relationships in working with schizophrenic patients. This chapter was originally a paper presented as part of a program titled "The Need for Innovative Treatments." Unfortunately, innovative psychosocial treatment is an oxymoron. Relational treatments, in fact, are the oldest we have. They predate the specific technical innovations of the past two generations about which we have heard so much in recent times. What is innovative about relationship treatments today is the urgent need we have to reassess and reassert their relevance and worth, because I am afraid that we have become a society greatly out of touch with our wish and capacity to care.

The terms "relationships" and "psychosocial forces" are used synonymously in this chapter. The review presented here is broad in scope, including a discussion of 1) psychosocial forces that have a demonstrated impact upon the natural history of schizophrenia and 2) the outcome dimensions of particular relevance for psychosocial treatments and psychosocial treatment research. After more closely examining one of these treatments, which has undergone the greatest innovation in the past decade, I conclude with some thoughts about three key historical landmarks in the psychosocial care and treatment of mentally ill people in America.

Psychosocial Forces and the Vicissitudes of Schizophrenia

How do psychosocial factors relate to the etiology and pathogenesis of schizophrenia? The question about etiology is the easiest to deal with; quite simply, such a role remains to be demonstrated. On the other hand, although the etiologic significance of nurture remains to be demonstrated, recent studies identify environmental factors as central to the pathogenesis and course of schizophrenia. This section will review studies of adoption, social class and culture, social networks, life events, and family factors.

Adoption Studies

Tienari et al. (1985) compared adopted-away children of schizophrenic mothers (probands) with adopted-away children of nonschizophrenic parents (control subjects). They replicated prior adoption study findings of a genetic link between schizophrenic probands and biological relatives. However, the nature of the rearing environment proved significant, as well. For example, *none* of 43 probands (children genetically at risk) raised in a relatively normal adoptive family environment met the criteria for psychosis or borderline personality disorder. In contrast, 15 of 39 probands (38%) raised in a severely disturbed adoptive family environment received one of these diagnoses. The authors formulated a hypothesis that a genetically transmitted vulnerability may be a necessary precondition for schizophrenia, but a distressing environment (here the family milieu) may also be necessary to transform the vulnerability into the overt syndrome.

Socioeconomic and Cultural Factors

Socioeconomic and cultural factors have a long empirical history of association with schizophrenia. One of the most replicated findings in the schizophrenia literature is the clustering of schizophrenic patients in the lowest social classes, especially in urban communities. Downward drift and selection account for much of this finding. Furthermore, the conditions of living at the lowest socioeconomic strata limit one's opportunities for coping resourcefully, thus elevating stress levels and symptomatic exacerbation in vulnerable individuals (Liberman 1982).

International follow-up data suggest a more benign course for schizophrenic patients in agrarian countries. Insofar as agrarian societies selectively apply therapeutic resources to more visible and floridly psychotic schizophrenic individuals with a better prognosis, this finding may reflect sampling artifact. Alternatively, it may reflect that more rural and economically primitive cultures confront vulnerable individuals with fewer demands for initiative and competitiveness, while providing them with tighter, smaller, and more enduring social and kinship networks (Strauss and Carpenter 1981).

Social Networks

Schizophrenia and social network are highly interactive cross-sectionally and longitudinally. Schizophrenic individuals usually have social networks that are smaller, less interconnected, simpler, more dependent, more casual and nonintimate, and more peopled with family as opposed to peers, than do nonschizophrenic individuals (Beels et al. 1984). The most dramatic changes in this direction follow the first hospitalization for schizophrenia. After three or more hospitalizations, families tend to disengage from the patient. A symptomatic episode forces temporary reliance upon dense formal network clusters (family, hospital, or clinic) requiring little initiative or exchange. Restoration to status before illness, when achieved, proceeds through formal transitional network clusters, such as churches, self-help groups, sheltered workshops, and day hospitals, where disability and poor motivation are not a bar to membership.

The interplay between schizophrenia and social networks appear to be circular rather than linear. Initially the major vector is schizophrenia upon social network. Following the appearance of clinical symptoms, however, social network is likely to exert a powerful influence upon the subsequent vicissitudes of schizophrenia.

Life Events

Stressful life events have a demonstrated association with schizophrenia, but this association may not always be necessary or direct. Questions often arise concerning whether stress differs in its effect upon disease onset versus recurrence, and whether a stressful event precedes illness or represents a product of symptom exacerbation.

Convention dichotomizes stressful events into those that are ambient, nonindependent, or chronic, versus those that are independent or acute. The former are stresses associated with everyday living, such as family, work, poverty, physical disability, and mental deficit; the latter are stresses associated with largely external and/or unusual changes, such as loss, death, acute illness, and relocations, especially if these changes are unanticipated, undesired, and uncontrolled. Research suggests a high frequency of such acutely stressful events shortly before schizophrenia onset or symptom exacerbation.

There also appears to be an important interaction between maintenance neuroleptic medication and life event stress. Patients in the community without medication are vulnerable to acute as well as chronic stress. Patients taking medication, however, appear to be protected against either type of stress, but are likely to relapse if *both* types occur together (Lukoff et al. 1984).

Family Factors

Potent interactions occur among certain family function dimensions and schizophrenic psychopathology. Three dimensions that have been operationalized and investigated are expressed emotion, affective style, and communication deviance.

Expressed emotion represents critical and/or emotionally over-involved attitudes and behaviors displayed by one or both parents toward their schizophrenic offspring. Families scoring high on this dimension also talk significantly more than low expressed emotion families. Expressed emotion is not specific to schizophrenia and is not necessarily pathogenic, especially in offspring without vulnerability to mental illness.

Affective style combines four parental attitudes and behaviors: criticism, guilt induction, intrusiveness, and inadequate support. Expressed emotion and affective style are interrelated (Goldstein 1984a).

Communication deviance includes parental communications that lack commitment to ideas and percepts; parental communications that are unclear because they are filled with idiosyncratic themes and ideas and have language anomalies, discursive speech, and problems with closure; and parental communications that reflect an inability to establish or maintain a shared focus of attention during transactions with another family member. This pattern is not specific to schizophrenia.

Doane et al. (1981) investigated communication deviance and affective style in 65 families with nonpsychotic but disturbed (at-risk) index adolescents. Independent systematic diagnosis 5 years later identified schizophrenic spectrum disorders among index cases and siblings. A significantly higher frequency of spectrum disorders was found in families with high affective style and communication deviance, compared with families with low affective style and communication deviance. A 15-year follow-up of the same family cohort using DSM-III criteria (American Psychiatric Association 1980), a tighter definition of the schizophrenia spectrum, and the additional family measure of expressed emotion essentially replicated the earlier finding (Goldstein 1984b). Four cases of schizophrenia were identified, all of whom came from families with moderate to high communication deviance, high expressed emotion, and negative affective style.

The expressed emotion variable bears significantly on the course of schizophrenia. British investigators (Leff and Vaughn 1981) found that schizophrenic patients discharged to high expressed emotion families relapsed within 9 months four times as frequently as schizophrenic patients returning to low expressed emotion families. Neuroleptic medication status and amount of weekly face-to-face contact between the index patient and his or her family further affected relapse rates among schizophrenic patients in high expressed emotion families as follows:

- High contact/no drug = 92% relapse
- High contact/drug = 53% relapse
- Low contact/no drug = 42% relapse
- Low contact/drug = 15% relapse

The higher frequency of relapse for high expressed emotion patients held at 2-year follow-up, although the prophylactic effect of maintenance drugs was no longer evident. Comparative relapse rates between high and low expressed emotion patients could not be attributed to differences in premorbid social adjustment, symptom severity, or chronicity.

These 9-month follow-up findings were replicated in a California sample, with the only difference being that medications protected high expressed emotion patients from relapse *only* if they also had low face-to-face contact (Vaughn et al. 1984). Results from Pittsburgh replicated the expressed emotion–relapse relationships, but only for a specific subgroup of patients who were male, younger, and more purely schizophrenic, as opposed to those who were schizoaffective and more severely ill at discharge (Hogarty 1984).

More recent work (Falloon 1988) suggests that what is pathogenic is not the presence of high expressed emotion, but the relative absence of low expressed emotion. For example, in low expressed emotion families, the relapse rate doubles when there is *less* face-to-face contact between patient and family members. This suggests that the quality of interpersonal support provided by the family or by professionals during aftercare may be crucially associated with clinical outcome and that the protective effects of stable, low expressed emotion environments and relationships may hold more clinical significance.

Overall, these studies demonstrate the heavy impact of psychosocial factors on the course of schizophrenia. The findings support the vulnerability-stress model of schizophrenia, which frequently serves as the basis for current thinking regarding psychosocial treatment intervention.

The Vulnerability-Stress Model

The vulnerability-stress model is a biopsychosocial model that accepts that the role of nurture in etiology will remain obscure until we have markers for the genetic predisposition or constitutional vulnerability to schizophrenia. The model shifts emphasis from the role of psychosocial factors in etiology to their role in facilitating and preventing the expression of the disease process (Spring and Zubin 1977).

The vulnerability to schizophrenia is seen as a relatively enduring proclivity toward developing clinical symptoms. It is a stable trait independent of non-enduring psychopathological states, meaning that its features are present premorbidly, at onset, during symptomatic efflorescence, and in remission. This trait should not, however, be regarded as developmentally static or fixed. Rather, it is shaped epigenetically via transactions with the environment at each developmental phase. Aspects of vulnerability are undoubtedly genetic. Some may be acquired biologically through intrauterine, birth, and postnatal complications. The evidence for psychosocially acquired vulnerability is meager at present, but cannot be ruled out (Wynne 1978).

The "stress" side of this model postulates that a variety of stressors, that is, internal or external events requiring adaptation, can convert vulnerability into symptoms. Therefore, coping strengths or supports that diminish stress should ameliorate or prevent the clinical expression of vulnerability.

The list of specific vulnerabilities is extensive. A few have been demonstrated, and many are postulated (Nuechterlein and Dawson 1984). First, there are deficits in the processing of complex information, in maintaining a steady focus of attention, in distinguishing between relevant and irrelevant stimuli, and in forming consistent abstractions. Second, there are dysfunctions in psychophysiology, suggesting deficits in sensory inhibition and poor control over autonomic responsivity, especially to aversive stimuli. Third, there are impairments in social competence, such as processing interpersonal stimuli, eye contact, assertiveness, or conversational capacity. These deficits probably reflect both a core disturbance of schizophrenia (vulnerability) and the social outcomes of severe psychopathology. In the past, the source of these difficulties was often attributed to such external elements as drugs or institutions, a perspective that unduly diverted attention from their primacy in the disorder. Fourth, there are general coping deficits, such as overevaluating threat, underappraising internal resources, or extensive use of denial.

Following the model, the vicissitudes of schizophrenia are determined by the nature of vulnerability and stress on the one hand, and the individual's strengths and environmental supports on the other. The interaction of sufficient stress with sufficient vulnerability can lead to transient intermediate (prodromal) states of dysfunction that amplify existing cognitive, affective-autonomic, and social-coping deficits. This compromised function in turn interacts negatively with stressors and magnifies their effect in a downwardly spiraling helical deterioration that ultimately bottoms out as a full-blown clinical syndrome.

The vulnerability-stress model can integrate the complex array of forces contributing to the heterogeneous long-term course and outcome of schizophrenia. Systematic investigations of longitudinal course have begun (Strauss et al. 1985), and a few clear and clinically familiar patterns have emerged. The most striking pattern concerns the *phasic* nature of recompensation.

Most schizophrenic patients progress from the active clinical state through a subacute phase of waning positive symptoms, into a period of postpsychotic depression, including sealing-over or conservation-withdrawal, during which they are markedly defensive, nonfunctional, and particularly vulnerable to symptom exacerbation under stress. From this phase they often progress to a phase of relative stability, or "moratorium," which may allow them to slowly reconstitute identity, accumulate supports, and strengthen skills. It may also, however, consolidate into a minimally adaptive chronic residual end state (McGlashan 1982). Further change during a moratorium, when it occurs, often happens quickly and unexpectedly. Such "change periods" are regularly accompanied by mild symptom exacerbations, which may progress to decompensation or resolve as the patient "integrates" at a new level of adaptation. The final

end state represents the denouement of this process. The resultant "outcomes" can vary enormously, from return to premorbid functioning, to
continuous disability.

A Natural History Perspective

Because the heterogeneity of schizophrenia is so vast, the long-term longitudinal or natural history perspective must be taken into account for
considerations of treatment and research. Across the entire range of
schizophrenic individuals, natural history may vary as shown in Figure
11–1. Outcome ranges from chronic disability to stable remission, and
these developments can be anticipated by the well-known predictors of
outcome of schizophrenia. Thus, the hypothetical "natural history" of
schizophrenia is different for each individual, depending on the balance of vulnerabilities, strengths, stresses, and supports. It is vital to be
aware of this profile because therapeutic change, as illustrated in Figure

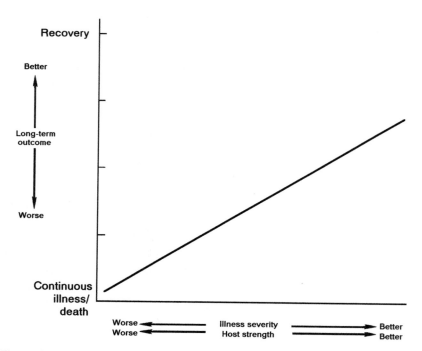

Figure 11–1. The natural history of schizophrenia: prognostic factors and
outcome.

11–2, must be measured against the long-term expectable baseline. It is also vital because the potential for change itself depends upon the baseline. With schizophrenia, as with all mental illness, we can expect more therapeutic gain in healthier patients.

This perspective also underscores that there is another level, the end containing severely mentally ill individuals, who are essentially untreatable—if by treatment we mean progress. This other end of the natural history regression line, the end of the chronically regressed, calls into question what is meant by treatment. What about services to those who cannot change or get better, that is, custodial services? Are those individuals to be ignored? To do so assumes that doing nothing is harmless and preserves the status quo. However, this may be far from the truth. As illustrated in Figure 11–3, although many of the severely mentally ill may not be able to get better, they can still get *worse*—as witnessed by our current tragedy of homelessness. In this context, custodial, or asylum, services, are decidedly active treatment, because they prevent deteriora-

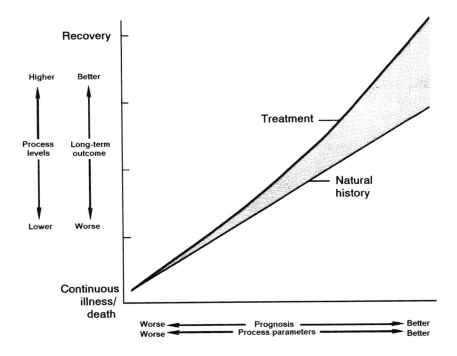

Figure 11–2. Treatment effect and natural history.

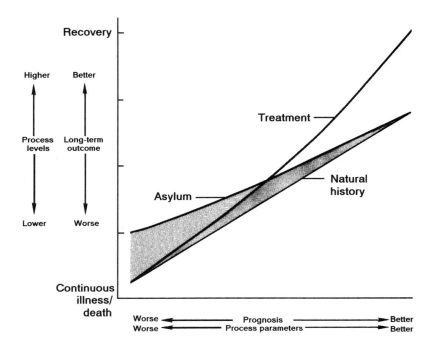

Figure 11–3. Asylum and treatment effect.

tion to a worse natural history baseline.

Therefore, our definition of psychosocial services must also include asylum services—supportive, custodial, holding services—and they should receive equal if not greater attention than the so-called active psychosocial therapeutic interventions. These asylum services are not popular either within the helping profession, because they are considered "therapeutically nihilistic," or outside of the profession, because they are expensive and ruin any "cost-effectiveness" advantage on the ledger sheets.

Outcome Dimensions Relevant to Psychosocial Treatment and Research

The regressed end of the regression line demands that we reconsider and expand what we regard as our treatment or service goals. Hargreaves and Shumway (1989) provided a starting point in defining these goals.

For mental health target populations, there are four relevant domains of service goals. They might be called clinical, rehabilitative, humanistic, and public safety goals. Clinical goals are to improve or cure an illness or disorder, reducing or eliminating its signs and symptoms. Rehabilitative goals are to restore or improve social and vocational functioning. Humanistic goals are to maximize patients' and family members' senses of well being and personal fulfillment. Public safety goals are to prevent injury to others and to patients, whether from assaultive or self-destructive behaviors that arise out of the illness, or from destructive side effects of the services themselves.

These four domains—clinical, rehabilitative, humanitarian, and public safety—cover most if not all of the outcomes relevant to mental illness and health. Each domain contains multiple dimensions, as elaborated in the following sections.

The Clinical Domain

The clinical outcome dimensions include various aspects of syndromal psychopathology and the course of these phenomenologies over time. These dimensions frequently include signs and symptoms, their aggregation into diagnostic entities, the amount and severity of symptomatology, and the amount and intensity of interventions required to control and/or treat these manifestations of illness (e.g., hospitalization, medication, types and amount of aftercare utilization).

Clinical outcome dimensions have been the most studied among the four domains in question. They are both categorical (e.g., diagnosis) and dimensional (e.g., severity of thought disorder) in nature. Many reliable and useful assessment instruments now exist to measure this vast array of dimensions, ranging from structured diagnostic interviews to dimensional rating scales. In fact, at this point it appears that clinical outcome assessment enjoys a surfeit of attention and instrumentation, and that initiatives for further development may best be targeted more toward other outcome domains.

The Rehabilitative Domain

Rehabilitation focuses on adaptation and functional capacity as opposed to illness and psychopathology. Rehabilitation strategies target a patient's strengths, existing talents, and coping strategies with which to minimize disability. Two broad outcome realms are relevant: social functioning and instrumental functioning.

Social functioning outcome dimensions are varied and include frequency of interpersonal contacts, closeness of these contacts, and degree of involvement in a meaningful social network, be it connected with work, school, family, peer group, or community support network. Implicit in these dimensions are constructs as basic as primitive social skills or as advanced as capacity for generativity. The marital status and parental status of patients reveal a great deal about their capacity for intimacy and the complexities of which they are capable in interpersonal relationships.

Patients with severe mental illness are very compromised socially. Their relationships, when they exist at all, are fleeting, superficial, exploitative, and suffused with conflict and anxiety. Yet many chronic patients meander within a loosely knit social network of similarly disenfranchised peers. Surprisingly, these networks are often quite sustaining and meaningful. Studies of the nature, constitution, creation, and evolution of these networks should be supported because, in addition to family and treatment network, these networks *are* the patient's community. The existence of these networks also helps make self-help organizations possible.

Instrumental functioning outcome dimensions encompass patients' problem-solving capacities, their ability to learn and to work, and the amount of initiative, drive, and frustration tolerance they bring to these pursuits. These outcome variables are among the most straightforward vis-à-vis ease of assessment. As outlined by Dion and Anthony (1987), for example, relevant measures include level of education (grade level, courses completed, degrees received, grades achieved, achievement test scores, etc.), level of employment (sheltered to competitive, part-time to full-time), level of work complexity (often reflected in earnings), productivity, satisfaction, and perseverance.

Perhaps the most uniform consequence of severe mental illness is a vastly compromised capacity for productive activity. If there is *any* pathognomonic sign of schizophrenia, it is unemployment. Virtually all psychotic patients are unable to work at some time, and the vast majority of chronically psychotic patients are unable to work all of the time—at least in competitive employment. For these patients, vocational rehabilitation efforts are always welcome, but for most of them the outcome cannot be described in the parlance of the usual marketplace. For the severely mentally ill, sheltered employment is required, either as practice in a transitional program or as the level of work of which the patient is maximally capable. To my knowledge, relevant measures of varying levels of sheltered work have not been devised, perhaps out of resistance to the idea that for many severely mentally ill patients these programs constitute end states: they are not transitional, but permanent.

The Humanitarian Domain

Humanitarian outcome dimensions are the least developed because humanitarian goals for the severely mentally ill are the most neglected. The presence of thousands of mentally ill homeless bears grim witness that we have abandoned humanitarian goals altogether. The causes of this appalling neglect are many and have been well delineated by E. F. Torrey (personal communication to the Clinical Services Research Panel, 1989).

Unfortunately, psychiatric research as interpreted by society has aided this neglect by abetting our denial about the reality of mental illness. The clear therapeutic advance documented by clinical trials of chlorpromazine was hailed as a cure and initiated the release of patients from state institutions. Since the 1970s, clinical service research studies have demonstrated repeatedly that shorter and less elaborate treatment programs do as well as their longer and more traditional counterparts vis-à-vis clinical and rehabilitative outcomes. This finding has been interpreted almost uniformly (quite gleefully by state legislators) as "less is just as good." This, in turn, has provided the rationale for wholesale cutbacks in state funding for our mentally indigent in the public sector. The *accurate* interpretation of these studies is actually tragic: they demonstrate that the illness wins again and again and that nothing really makes any difference. Upholding the null hypothesis about comparative service interventions, however, has been taken to mean that mental disability is null and nonexistent.

Future clinical services research must address this denial, in part by asserting, nonapologetically, that there are very real limits to our therapeutic strategies with the severely mentally ill *and* that humanitarian considerations demand that we provide supportive asylum at the boundaries of these limits. The nature of this asylum is only beginning to be articulated in our society's consciousness. Clearly the old-time state institution is dead and community mental health care is here to stay. What we want as helping professionals also seems clear: the severely mentally ill patient receiving good enough clinical care (for clinical outcomes) and realistic rehabilitation efforts (for rehabilitative outcomes), *and* receiving all the supports and shelters in the community that he or she would have received in a *good* state hospital system 40 years ago.

Future clinical services research must help articulate the humanitarian outcomes, that is, the structural and functional specifics of community asylum. Some of these specifics are clear, at least in principle: adequate food, clothing, and shelter. Other questions require careful study, such as how to maximize a patient's self-care capacities, how to recognize the limitations of these capacities in a patient, how then to tailor a living situation that matches these limitations, and how providing such a match affects a patient's well-being and quality of life.

Subjective well-being and quality of life constitute the ultimate humanitarian goals, and a few relevant instruments exist to assess these dimensions. However, they need to be elaborated to match the depth and complexity of severe mental illness. For example, what constitutes optimal, subjective well-being in a patient with chronic (and treatment-resistant) hallucinosis, or what type of extrafamilial living situation (if any) maximizes the quality of life for a chronically dependent patient with deficit schizophrenia living with an overburdened family?

In addition to the technical task of developing realistic and relevant humanitarian outcome instruments, the primary importance of humanitarian goals must be recognized. At the very least, humanitarian dimensions should be included in every study that also measures cost an as outcome variable. It is time for the services research community to test and challenge the assumption that "cheaper is better" by documenting the actual relationships between price of service and quality of life. Such research is vital to guide our society in forging newer, more enlightened community-based asylums for our severely mentally ill.

The Public Safety Domain

When we declared our independence as a nation, we did so to pursue and to guarantee the "inalienable" human rights of life, liberty, and the pursuit of happiness. Having achieved some maturity and a measure of wisdom over two centuries, we can recognize that these rights are not always complementary. In particular, our recent preoccupation with individual civil liberties, at least for many of the homeless mentally ill individuals, has occasionally endangered life and has regularly compromised the pursuit of happiness by allowing patients who are incapable of realistic planning to reconnoiter by themselves. As such, judgmental paralytics are "set free," and, like ships without rudders, they meander forth from the harbor of paternalism—free but helpless, rotting with their rights on.

The network of clinical services to the severely mentally ill has watched with equal helplessness as the legal juggernaut has systematically stripped paternalism of its clout. However, the unhealthy result of this preoccupation with liberty is abundantly apparent on our nation's streets, heating grates, and bus and train stations. Now patients can be committed to treatment services only if they are extremely and imminently dangerous to themselves or society. By shackling reasonable coercion to this degree, the civil libertarians have created a much larger and more insidious danger to the patient's life and pursuit of happiness.

It is time for the clinical services community to actively challenge the assumptions that liberty is sacred above all. It is time to confront the legal profession and demand a whole new frontier of research—that of the consequences (clinical, rehabilitative, humanitarian) of differing civil commitment statutes. Public safety outcome dimensions should no longer be restricted to frequency of assaultive and/or self-destructive behaviors. They should be expanded to include physical safety (right to life) and psychological well-being (right to happiness). The current ideational hegemony that these rights are guaranteed by liberty has yet to be tested scientifically. The legal profession needs to be informed beyond its adversarial polemics, because the civil liberty statutes are based upon the assumption of intact judgmental capacity; in other words, they are constructed upon blatant denial of mental illness. Only careful research can definitively challenge this denial.

As a beginning, perhaps, we need to reassess our latter-day alliance with the public service accountants. I submit that cost-effectiveness as a primary psychosocial outcome measure is a red herring. Considerations of cost have accrued far too much power in comparative studies of clinical treatment services delivery, perhaps because money spent is the easiest outcome variable to measure. But now cost must take its place within the matrix of multidimensionality. For example, linkage with viable aftercare services constitutes the optimal outcome for many patients with severe mental illness upon discharge from a hospital, but such an outcome is hardly cost-effective compared with total disengagement. If cost of services is to be measured in future comparative treatment studies, the cost to patients, to their families, and to society of the *absence* or *refusal* of services must also be estimated and factored in. We must tell the accountants that the alternatives to institutionalization are equally if not more expensive.

Psychosocial Treatments for Schizophrenia: General Considerations

Treatment Principles

The current psychosocial treatments of schizophrenia reflect a shift toward pragmatism, efficacy testing, and community locus. They share the following principles that are common to virtually all forms of treatment of schizophrenia:

1. Schizophrenia is heterogeneous, as are the individuals afflicted with it. Because of this, *there is no single or preferred treatment.* Instead, schizophrenia requires a broad approach with multiple therapies applied in varying sequence, depending upon the nature and phase of illness, environmental circumstances, and individual assets and weaknesses. The ongoing aim is to maximize the ratio of strength and support, rather than vulnerability and stress, by treating disease, minimizing stress, mobilizing resources, and salvaging and rehabilitating healthy ego functions.
2. The core of treatment is the clinical relationship: the interpersonal context, with the professional extensively and emphatically involved as a participant-observer.
3. Treatment must be consistent, must be temporally open-ended (perhaps lifelong), and must offer continuity of treating persons, teams, or institutions.
4. Therapists should, ideally, be resistant to premature closure, yet willing to act when necessary despite inadequate information; be flexible, avoid polarized thinking, and recognize commonalities among treatments; be humble, reality oriented, and receptive of help and outside support; be patient with and tolerant of psychopathology, negativism, and deficits, without losing optimism on the one hand, or becoming too zealous therapeutically on the other; and be respectful of the patient's humanity, privacy, autonomy, and need for distance (McGlashan 1983).

General Treatment Strategies

A number of strategies are common to all of the psychosocial treatments under consideration. The first common strategy is *evaluation.* A thorough evaluation of the patient initiates the process of treatment. Especially important is ruling out disorders with other treatment implications.

The second common strategy is *continuous reevaluation*. The dynamic and fluid nature of schizophrenia demands periodic reassessment of course and prognosis, phase of illness, and target problems. As these change, so do treatment goals. A low expressed emotion family, for example, may be therapeutic during the acute phase of illness, but may foster deficit functioning later on.

The third common strategy is *timing*. Consideration of the phasic nature of schizophrenic episodes dictates that attention be paid to when certain treatments are indicated. According to Hogarty (1984), for example, little if anything should be expected of the patient for the first 6 to 12 months following an episode, to minimize stress and forestall relapse. Once the patient is asymptomatic and shows the first signs of revitalization, rehabilitation efforts may be introduced slowly, with only one thing being changed at a time. Higher levels of nonsheltered social and/or instrumental functioning are attempted 1–2 years later, but only upon completion and consolidation of earlier gains.

The fourth common strategy is *titration*. Treatments should be applied with graded increases in intensity and complexity. There is evidence that early, active, and ambitious psychosocial treatments may be toxic for certain patients (Liberman 1982). This does *not* endorse a treatment strategy of withdrawal and neglect, but highlights the importance of tailoring and titrating treatment interventions.

The final common strategy is *integration with psychopharmacology*. The new psychosocial treatments take neuroleptic drugs as given and formulate integrated strategies that are aimed at optimizing the therapeutic effects and minimizing the side effects of both. Some psychosocial programs (e.g., social learning and/or token economy) have proved most useful in intractable, chronic patients who are free of medication. Most studies, however, find that drugs and psychosocial programs have a positive association, either additive or interactive (Falloon and Liberman 1983).

Phase-Specific Strategies

Although a comprehensive phase-specific system of treatment guidelines has yet to be articulated or tested, some component strategies have been offered.

Late prodromal and acute phase. Treatment goals in this phase are to prevent harm, control disturbed behavior, suppress symptoms, effect a rapid return to the best level of functioning, forge an alliance with the patient and family, devise a long-term treatment plan, and link the patient with appropriate continuity of care. This requires hospitalization or a safe alternate facility in the community. The milieu must set firm limits and use seclusion if necessary. Neuroleptic medications are the rule. Psychosocial interventions aim at reducing stimuli and promoting relaxation through simple, clear, coherent communications and expectations, a structured environment, low performance requirements, and tolerant, nondemanding, supportive relationships.

Subacute phase and postpsychotic depression. The principal goal here is to prevent relapse. Drugs are continued. Psychosocial interventions remain supportive and nondemanding, and they are usually less coercive. Now, however, the patient is home, which necessitates family education, management, and therapy, because the family constitutes the milieu. More engaging or ambitious psychosocial treatments, such as intensive psychotherapy, insight-oriented group therapy, or vocational rehabilitation, are held in abeyance.

Moratorium or adaptive plateau. The primary goal during this phase is, at the least, to lock the patient into a stable (albeit suboptimal) adaptive plateau or, at the most, to restore the patient to his or her most effective level of functioning. The patient is usually still living at home. Once the patient becomes asymptomatic and relatively motivated, supportive but more systematic psychosocial treatment strategies can be introduced, such as reeducation in basic living skills, social skills training, and rudimentary vocational rehabilitation. Supportive, structured extrafamilial groups are encouraged for social contact. If the treatment alliance is sufficiently robust so that the patient or family can identify and report prodromal symptoms, drug dosage may be reduced or targeted drug strategies instituted.

Change periods. The phenomenology and dynamics of change periods have yet to be described. Treatment strategies are therefore speculative at best. Careful observation and close but nonintrusive "hovering" may be needed during this period of disequilibrium—coupled with a readiness for crisis intervention if the phasic momentum veers toward relapse instead of reintegration.

End states. The goals here are to prevent relapse, to maintain the patient at an optimal level of functioning and, if possible, to foster progress in the realms of emotional maturity, social affinity, and instrumental proclivity. For patients with minimal deficit symptoms, psychosocial interventions such as group or family therapy can be more complex, ambitious, and demanding, especially if drugs are used in a buffered capacity. Patients with marked deficit states, however, require a return to the earlier more structured, supportive, and soothing psychosocial strategies.

Deficits, by definition, imply greater or lesser degrees of functional paralysis. Accordingly, provision must be made for asylum. Treatment providers and family need to recognize that limits exist to the patient's capacities and that he or she may be dependent upon others prosthetically for a lifetime. Each deficit syndrome is, to some extent, a one-way street requiring unidirectional expenditures in time and energy. This should be expected, and the treatment system should be so constructed that sufficient resources and supports can be provided to patients, family, and treating staff, *indefinitely*. Without this, bitterness, burnout, and ultimate neglect of these patients become inevitable.

Family Therapy

Many specific psychosocial treatments are available, including milieu therapy, behavior therapy, social and vocational skills training, group therapy, and family therapy. All of them are important, but our focus will be only on family therapy, because it has undergone the most change since the early 1980s, and its transformations have richly informed us about how to structure changes in other psychosocial treatments.

In one decade, family therapy for schizophrenia has leaped forward as *the* psychosocial modality of greatest interest. Partly this stems from need: that is, community treatment relies heavily upon families as the new therapeutic milieu. Partly this stems from a new attitude of respect for these families. This attitude makes collaboration with mental health professionals more palatable. Mostly, however, interest exists because these methods have repeatedly proved to be *effective* in well-designed clinical trials.

Almost without exception, these "new" family therapies endorse and build their technical strategies around the vulnerability-stress model of schizophrenia. Families are not regarded as "causing" schizophrenia, but are seen as capable of profoundly affecting its onset and course, especially in a positive direction in collaboration with professional help. Treatment goals are more modest and pragmatic than they were in the past: amelioration of the course of illness, not cure; diminished relapse beyond that produced by prophylactic medication alone; and enhanced psychosocial functioning and integration into the community.

Several formats of family therapy have evolved; they are adequately described elsewhere (McFarlane 1983). Most contain such technical elements as joining with family members in an empathic, nonblaming alliance; psychoeducation about schizophrenia and its management; identification of prodromal signs of relapse for targeting drug interventions; training in changing maladaptive interaction patterns such as expressed emotion, negative affective style, and communication deviance; reducing stigmatization; and expanding social networks.

Table 11–1 presents the relapse rates for three different family therapy programs. The numbers speak for themselves. The group from Pittsburgh found that patient stabilization and functional gains took far longer to achieve than anticipated—usually approximately 2 years following hospitalization. They also concluded that their individual family sessions were too frequent (and therefore pressuring). Crises were fewer and compliance with treatment aims was better when the weekly sessions were reduced to every other week.

Goldstein (1984a) suggests that this kind of family therapy not be used in the acute first break situation, when diagnosis and prognosis are ambiguous and patients and families are not motivated for the necessary

Table 11–1.   Relapse rate and family treatments

Study	N	Follow-up period	Family therapy	Family therapy and social skills training	Social skills training	Drugs only
Falloon et al. 1982 (California)	36	9 months	6	—	—	44
Leff et al. 1982 (Britain)	24	9 months	9	—	—	50
Hogarty et al. 1991 (Pittsburgh)	90	1 year	19	0	20	38

long-term effort. He also suggests that the primary impact of psycho-education is more attitudinal than education per se. Families are more realistic about what to expect from treatment and feel they have allies in the mental health profession.

Historical Landmarks of Psychosocial Treatment in America

I wish to conclude with a survey of what I consider to be the major his-torical landmarks of psychosocial treatments of the severely mentally ill in America. I do this out of a conviction that the true innovations in our relationship therapies represent but rediscoveries of our common human legacy, as witnessed and articulated by three pivotal forebears: Dorothea Dix, Harry Stack Sullivan, and George Brooks.

In 1841, a 32-year-old Sunday School teacher was riveted by the sight of a madwoman bound by chains to the walls of a jail. Thus began Doro-thea Dix's lifelong crusade to bring moral treatment to the mentally ill in America, to release them from their societal stigma and remove them to institutional asylums. Her effort was motivated by the conviction that if insanity was detected soon enough, and its victims treated with kindness and dignity, they would recover in weeks or months, as if they were suffer-ing from a cold or the flu. Her lobbying efforts in Washington and with Presidents Fillmore and Lincoln were ultimately responsible for the con-struction of 32 asylums—communities set apart where the mentally ill could be removed from stress and from the punitive eyes of the public.

Unfortunately, her therapeutic vision proved to be naive. The insane could be released from societal chains, but not from the chains of illness. Most of those housed in the asylums proved to be suffering from chronic disorders, and they soon became warehoused and just as isolated in vitro as they had been in vivo. By the turn of the century, state hospitals came to be viewed phobically as Victorian houses of horror—blessedly removed to purgatorial memorial parks beyond the community.

Into the midst of this standoff walked a young psychiatrist who car-ried with him the conviction that the insane are more human than oth-erwise and that they possess a potential for health. Harry Stack Sullivan created a truly innovative inpatient ward for acutely ill, male schizophren-ic patients at Sheppard and Enoch Pratt Hospital in Towson, Maryland, in the 1920s. It was the first of its kind in the world in its use of enlight-ened milieu treatment, in its use of pharmacotherapy for the acute phase of psychosis, and in its use of interpersonal psychotherapy, or talking to patients as human beings.

Sullivan outlined this approach in a talk to the American Psychiatric Association at its meeting in Toronto in 1931 (Sullivan 1931). About the use of structured milieu, he said:

> The procedure of treatment begins with removing the patient from the situation in which he is developing difficulty, to a situation in which he is encouraged to renew efforts at adjustment with others. . . . The [para]professional with whom the patient is in contact must be aware of the principal difficulty, [that is] the extreme sensitivity underlying whatever camouflage the patient may use. They must be activated by a well integrated purpose of helping in the redevelopment or development, de novo, of self esteem as an individual attractive to others. They must possess sufficient insight into their own personality organization to be able to avoid masked or unconscious sadism, jealousies, and morbid expectations and results. . . . Admittedly, this is no small order, and the creation of this sort of situation is scarcely to be expected either from chance or from the efforts of a commonplace administrative agent.
>
> Given the therapeutic environment, the first stage of therapy by the physician takes the form of providing an orienting experience. After the initial, fairly searching interview, the patient is introduced to the new situation in a matter-of-fact fashion, with emphasis on the personal elements. In other words, he is made to feel he is now one of the group, composed partly of sick persons . . . and well folk. Emphasis is laid on the fact that something is the matter with the patient and . . . that regardless of the patient's occasional or habitual surmise to the contrary, everyone who is well enough to be a help will, from thence forth be occupied in giving him a chance to get well. From the start, he is treated as a person among persons.
>
> There is never to be either an acceptance of his disordered thought and behavior as crazy. . . . Everyone is to regard the outpouring of thought or the doing of acts as at least valid for the patient, and to be considered seriously as something that at least he should understand.

Sullivan's next comments were about the use of chemotherapy to quell acute agitation and foster socialization; keep in mind that this was the 1920s.

> If the patient does not respond in so gratifying a fashion to the special environment, the physician must discover the difficulty. In some cases, the previously dissociated tendency system is integrating personal situ-

ations that precipitate panic. [Here I think he is referring to patients who incorporate the milieu in their delusional systems and begin to experience the hospital in irrationally fearful ways.] In all too many cases [the environment] is judged by the [patient] to be ominous, and the attempt to diminish the violence of reaction . . . fails. It is necessary, however, that the conflict be abated, otherwise the development of interpersonal security that is absolutely necessary for recovery cannot be achieved. In such cases, resource is had to chemotherapeutic agencies, notably ethyl alcohol, which impair the highly discriminative action of lately acquired tendency symptoms, [i.e., disordered thinking] and permit the at least rudimentary functioning of the [more normal], without much stress. After from three to ten days of continuous, mild intoxication, almost all such patients, in the writer's experience, have effected a considerable readjustment. . . . These patients discover by actual experience that the personal environment is not noxious, and, having discovered this, have great difficulty in subsequently elaborating convictions of menace, plots, etc. It is the rule to have several interviews with the patient during the period of intoxication, and in them to carry out the reassuring technique above indicated.

And all of this was said in the context of Prohibition!

Finally, I sum Sullivan's comments on the use of talking treatment or interpersonal psychotherapy.

As the patient improves, and as his acceptance of the need for help grows, some of the efforts of the physician become more direct in their application. Energy is expended briefly in reconstructing the actual chronology of the psychosis. . . . The role of significant persons and their doings is emphasized, the patient being constantly under the influence of the formulation above set forth, that however mysteriously the phenomena originated, everything that has befallen him is related to actual living among a relatively small number of significant people, in a relatively simple course of events. Psychotic phenomena recalled from the more disturbed periods are subjected to study as to their relation to these people. . . . During this phase of the work, the patient may or may not grasp the dynamics of his difficulty as they become apparent to the physician. Interpretations are never to be forced on him, and preferably none are offered.

Sullivan brought the humane community to the hospital, and he did these things over 60 years ago. How often do we have to reinvent the wheel?

The next great leap forward took place about 30 years later in the quiet, rural setting of Waterbury, Vermont, at the Vermont State Hospital. A psychiatrist, George Brooks, who may well be America's Eugen or Manfred Bleuler, initiated the process of bringing the hospital back to the community. This program, like Sullivan's, was the first of its kind in many respects. It was the first, and for many years, the only program of community mental health and deinstitutionalization in America that *worked*. It was probably the first use of chemotherapy for maintenance purposes in aftercare, and it was undoubtedly the first treatment program organized around serious efforts at vocational rehabilitation. All of this is outlined in a relatively unknown document entitled "The Vermont Story" (Chittick et al. 1961).

The program began at Vermont State Hospital around 1955 in conjunction with the introduction of chlorpromazine in the United States. For those chronically institutionalized patients who were partial drug responders or who responded but remained de-skilled, a rehabilitation ward was constructed which included intensive milieu therapy in the Sullivan mode, vocational rehabilitation with an active work program in the hospital, and discharge from the hospital to preexisting transitional living facilities and to preexisting jobs within a receptive community. The patients were provided continuity of care coordinated and administered by the director, George Brooks, himself, for the next 25 to 30 years.

The remarkable thing is that even though this was the first such program in America, it has been, perhaps, the only one to avoid the countless pitfalls plaguing such efforts elsewhere around the country. The people in Vermont seemed to do everything right. In their maintenance chemotherapy, for example, they used a low-dose strategy. In the hospital they kept patients very busy, thus minimizing secondary gain. They pre-erected jobs and living facilities in the community and avoided what has become the major downfall of America's community mental health movement. And the program provided optimal continuity of care, not just of treating structure, but of treating persons as well.

The results of this endeavor are impressive. The long-term follow-up of these patients has been reported by Harding (1987a, 1987b). Although their outcome undoubtedly reflects sample characteristics, as I recently discussed (McGlashan 1988), the outcome also undoubtedly reflects their treatment program.

What is next? Dix *created* the promise of relationships by identifying the "different" as diseased, as humans in need of removal from stress—in need of asylum. Sullivan *revitalized* the promise of relationships by bringing community into the alienated mental institutions. Brooks *liberalized* the promise of relationships by moving the institutional residents back into the community. It was about 90 years from Dix to Sullivan, and another 30 to Brooks. It has been another 30-some years since then—years that have seen enlightenment struggle to stay alive despite these mentors, years that have seen deinstitutionalization uninformed by the experience at Vermont State Hospital; rather, years that have seen deinstitutionalization as a grand political football, deinstitutionalization as projectile vomiting of our disabled onto the sidewalks.

We have thrust the severely mentally ill out of the institutions only to forget the first lesson that Dorothea Dix taught us: they are disabled and they need asylum, in the sense of support and protection from stress. Waking up from Erving Goffman's *Asylum* nightmare or escaping from Ken Kesey's *One Flew Over the Cuckoo's Nest* prison does not liberate one from brain disease. Most severely mentally ill patients still need asylum in the community. Perhaps this can be our goal over the next 30 years. I am not really sure what will be our next great leap forward, but I do know one thing—we sure are ready for something because it sure is bad out there. We must approach this vacuum of caring in our traditional roles as clinicians and researchers, but also with stealth and resolve as political advocates.

References

American Psychiatric Association: Diagnostic and Statistical Manual of Mental Disorders, 3rd Edition. Washington, American Psychiatric Association, 1980

Beels CC, Gutwirth L, Berkeley J, et al: Measurements of social support in schizophrenia. Schizophr Bull 10:399–411, 1984

Chittick RA, Brooks GW, Irons FS, et al: The Vermont Story: Rehabilitation of Chronic Schizophrenic Patients. Burlington, VT, Queen City Printers, 1961

Dion GL, Anthony WA: Research in psychiatric rehabilitation: a review of experimental and quasi-experimental studies. Rehabilitation Counseling Bulletin 30:177–203, 1987

Doane JA, West KL, Goldstein MJ, et al: Parental communication deviance and affective style. Arch Gen Psychiatry 38:679–685, 1981

Falloon IRH: Expressed emotion: current status. Psychol Med 18:269–274, 1988

Falloon IRH, Liberman RP: Interactions between drug and psychosocial therapy in schizophrenia. Schizophr Bull 9:543–554, 1983

Falloon IRH, Boyd JL, McGill CW, et al: Family management in the prevention of exacerbations of schizophrenia: a controlled study. N Engl J Med 306:1437–1440, 1982

Goffman E: Asylums: essays on the social situation of mental patients and other inmates. Garden City, NY, Doubleday, 1961

Goldstein MJ: Family factors that antedate the onset of schizophrenia and related disorders: the results of a 15-year prospective longitudinal study. Paper presented at the Regional Symposium of the World Psychiatric Association, Helsinki, Finland, June 1984a

Goldstein MJ: Family intervention programs, in Schizophrenia Treatment, Management, and Rehabilitation. Edited by Bellack AS. Orlando, FL, Grune & Stratton, 1984b

Harding CM, Brooks GW, Ashikaga T, et al: The Vermont longitudinal study of persons with severe mental illness, I: methodology, study sample, and overall status 32 years later. Am J Psychiatry 144:718–726, 1987a

Harding CM, Brooks GW, Ashikaga T, et al: The Vermont longitudinal study of persons with severe mental illness, II: long-term outcome of subjects who retrospectively met DSM-III criteria for schizophrenia. Am J Psychiatry 144:727–735, 1987b

Hargreaves WA, Shumway M: Effectiveness of mental health services for the severely mentally ill, in The Future of Mental Health Services Research (National Institute of Mental Health; DHHS Publ No ADM-89-1600). Edited by Taube CA, Mechanic D, Hohmann A. Washington, DC, U.S. Government Printing Office, 1989

Hogarty GE: Depot neuroleptics: the relevance of psychosocial factors—a United States perspective. J Clin Psychiatry 45:36–42, 1984

Hogarty GE, Anderson CM, Reiss DJ, et al: Family psychoeducation, social skills training, and maintenance chemotherapy in aftercare treatment of schizophrenia. Arch Gen Psychiatry 48:340–347, 1991

Kesey K: One Flew Over the Cuckoo's Nest. New York, Penguin Books, 1962

Leff J, Vaughn C: The role of maintenance therapy and relatives' expressed emotion in relapse of schizophrenia: a two-year follow-up. Br J Psychiatry 139:102–104, 1981

Leff J, Kuipers L, Berkowitz R, et al: A controlled trial of social intervention in the families of schizophrenic patients. Br J Psychiatry 141:121–134, 1982

Liberman RP: Social factors in the etiology of the schizophrenic disorders, in Psychiatry 1982: The American Psychiatric Association Annual Review, Vol 1. Edited by Grinspoon L. Washington, DC, American Psychiatric Press, 1982

Lukoff D, Snyder K, Ventura J, et al: Life events, familial stress, and coping in the developmental course of schizophrenia. Schizophr Bull 10:258–292, 1984

McFarlane WR: Family Therapy in Schizophrenia. New York, Guilford, 1983

McGlashan TH: Aphanisis: the syndrome of pseudo-depression in chronic schizophrenia. Schizophr Bull 8:118–134, 1982

McGlashan TH: Intensive individual psychotherapy of schizophrenia: a review of techniques. Arch Gen Psychiatry 40:909–920, 1983

McGlashan TH: Selective review of recent North American long-term follow-up studies of schizophrenia. Schizophr Bull 14:515–542, 1988

Nuechterlein KH, Dawson ME: Vulnerability and stress factors in the developmental course of schizophrenic disorders. Schizophr Bull 10:158–159, 1984

Spring B, Zubin J: Vulnerability to schizophrenic episodes and their prevention in adults, in Primary Prevention in Psychopathology: The Issues, Vol 1. Edited by Albee GW, Joffee JM. Hanover, NH: University Press of New England, 1977

Strauss JS, Carpenter WT: Schizophrenia. New York, Plenum, 1981

Strauss JS, Hafez H, Liberman P, et al: The course of psychiatric disorder, III: longitudinal principles. Am J Psychiatry 142:289–296, 1985

Sullivan HS: The modified psychoanalytic treatment of schizophrenia. Am J Psychiatry 11:519–540, 1931

Tienari P, Sorri A, Lahti I, et al: The Finnish adoptive family study of schizophrenia. Yale J Biol Med 58:227–237, 1985

Vaughn CE, Snyder KS, Jones S, et al: Family factors in schizophrenic relapse: replication in California of British research on expressed emotion. Arch Gen Psychiatry 41:1169–1177, 1984

Wynne LC: From symptoms to vulnerability and beyond: an overview, in The Nature of Schizophrenia: New Approaches to Research and Treatment. Edited by Wynne LC, Cromwell RL, Matthysse S. New York, Wiley, 1978

Section V

A Glimpse of the Future

The Molecular Basis of Schizophrenia

Prologue to Section V

A Glimpse of the Future

The Molecular Basis of Schizophrenia

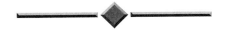

The identification of the double helix of DNA opened a new era for modern medicine. The breaking of the genetic code, when coupled with the newer techniques of molecular biology that permit receptor cloning and sophisticated linkage studies, offers the promise that we may identify the causes of diseases at the most basic level. That is, we can hope to understand how cells within the body and the brain are coded to send messages that produce dysfunctions in growth, metabolism, physiology, and biochemistry. These techniques have been used to understand a variety of medical disorders, such as Huntington's disease and muscular dystrophy.

This section contains two chapters about the efforts to apply insights at the molecular level to the study of mechanisms that produce schizophrenia. In Chapter 12, Dr. Jay W. Pettegrew and Dr. Nancy J. Minshew describe a method that integrates neuroradiology with the study of cell membrane function at the molecular level; specifically, the application of nuclear magnetic resonance spectroscopy to the study of cell membrane physiology in first-episode schizophrenic patients. They present findings suggesting that schizophrenic patients may have abnormalities in phospholipid metabolism in the prefrontal cortex; the changes observed are consistent with either abnormal patterns of brain development or acceleration of processes in the brain that occur during aging.

In Chapter 13, Dr. Raymond R. Crowe describes the application of the techniques of molecular genetics to the study of schizophrenia. He provides an overview of the recent revolution in molecular genetics, which has been made possible through the identification of restriction fragment length polymorphisms (RFLPs). He begins by describing the basic principles of these new molecular genetic techniques, including the study of candidate genes and linkage studies. He summarizes some of the recent efforts to find a linkage with chromosome 5 and schizophrenia, which have yielded conflicting and predominantly negative results. His thoughtful discussion of the challenges inherent in the application of molecular genetics provides a useful cautionary warning to those who hope that the riddle of schizophrenia will be solved quickly.

Schizophrenia is a complex illness at the clinical level, and it is no doubt highly complex at the level of pathophysiology and etiology. It probably represents a final common pathway that is produced by a variety of both genetic and environmental causes. Its heterogeneity has been the major obstacle that has prevented it from yielding its secrets to the many talented and persistent investigators who have pursued them up to this point. Nevertheless, as the various chapters in this book have indicated, enormous progress has been made in the study of schizophrenia. Clinicians and investigators now feel that they have many useful tools in hand, providing hope that we may achieve greater understanding, improved treatment, and perhaps ultimately prevention.

Chapter 12

Molecular Insights Into Schizophrenia

Jay W. Pettegrew, M.D.
Nancy J. Minshew, M.D.

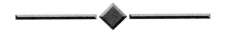

In this chapter we review the use of phosphorus-31 nuclear magnetic resonance (^{31}P NMR) to assess brain high-energy phosphate and membrane phospholipid metabolism. After a brief review of studies that have demonstrated alterations in the structure and function of the frontal cortex in some schizophrenic patients, we describe and compare in vitro and in vivo ^{31}P NMR studies. The findings of our study comparing 11 schizophrenic patients with 10 matched healthy control subjects are presented, and the implications of these findings for the pathogenesis and treatment of schizophrenia are discussed.

Michelle Young is gratefully acknowledged for typing the manuscript and for her helpful editorial assistance.

Evidence for Impaired Frontal Lobe Function and Membrane Alterations in Schizophrenia

Several lines of evidence indicate impaired frontal lobe function ("hypofrontality") in some schizophrenic patients (Buchsbaum et al. 1982; Weinberger et al. 1986). Cerebral blood flow studies using xenon-133 demonstrate a reduced ratio of frontal lobe to whole surface blood flow in schizophrenic patients under resting conditions (Ingvar and Franzen 1974) and during cortical activation with the Wisconsin Card Sorting Test (Berman et al. 1988; Heaton 1985). Reduced frontal-to-occipital metabolic rate also is observed in some schizophrenic patients (Buchsbaum 1987). These studies suggest that further metabolic studies of the frontal lobe might enhance our understanding of the pathophysiology of schizophrenia. Since normal brain function is dependent on normal high-energy phosphate and membrane phospholipid metabolism, either or both of these aspects of brain metabolism might be altered in schizophrenia.

Other evidence links possible membrane-related abnormalities to the pathophysiology of major psychoses. Several studies examining erythrocyte membrane phospholipids have shown phosphatidylcholine (PtdC) to be reduced in some patients with schizophrenia (Henn 1980; Hitzemann et al. 1984; Stevens 1972). Increases in phosphatidylserine (PtdS) and smaller decreases in phosphatidylethanolamine (PtdE) also have been noted, but less consistently replicated (Rotrosen and Wolkin 1987). Such abnormalities appear to be independent of previous drug treatment (Stevens 1972). Phospholipase A_2 activity, which alters phospholipid fatty acid composition through the deacylation-reacylation cycle, has been found to be increased in some schizophrenic patients (Gattaz et al. 1987). In addition, Kaiya et al. (1984) have described abnormalities in the phosphatidylinositol (PtdI) cycle in a subgroup of schizophrenic patients. There are, therefore, reasons to suspect alterations in brain membrane phospholipid metabolism in some patients with schizophrenia. However, to date, these parameters have been examined only in peripheral tissues. Support for drawing analogies between peripheral blood elements and brain tissue is derived from observed membrane abnormalities in peripheral cells in Huntington's chorea, myotonic dystrophy, affective illness, and Alzheimer's disease (Blass et al. 1985; Butterfield and Markesbery 1980; Butterfield et al. 1977, 1978, 1985; Diamond et al. 1983; Markesbery et al. 1980; Miller et al. 1989; Pettegrew et al. 1979a, 1979b, 1979c, 1981, 1982, 1983b; Sherman et al. 1986; Zubenko et al. 1987).

^{31}P NMR Assessment of Brain High-Energy Phosphate and Membrane Phospholipid Metabolism

In Vitro Studies

^{31}P NMR spectroscopy has proved to be a powerful analytical method for investigating phosphorus metabolism in neural and extraneural tissues (Barany and Glonek 1984). Studies on neural tissues have utilized tissue extracts (Glonek et al. 1982; Pettegrew et al. 1979b), in vitro brain slices (Cohen et al. 1984), and in vivo studies of animals and humans (Ackerman et al. 1980; Cady et al. 1983; Chance et al. 1978; Maris et al. 1985; Petroff et al. 1985).

In vitro analytical studies provide chemical conditions that are more favorable for ^{31}P NMR analysis than those occurring in the living brain and, therefore, achieve greater sensitivity and resolution. The enhanced sensitivity and resolution of in vitro extract studies allow the characterization and quantitation of many different phosphorus-containing compounds. Results from in vitro studies are very important to properly interpret in vivo findings in which the resolution and peak dispersion are reduced. Data from previous in vitro ^{31}P NMR studies demonstrated a remarkable correlation with those obtained from more classical assay procedures and, in addition, revealed previously uncharacterized metabolites and unrecognized metabolic relationships (Cohen et al. 1984; Glonek et al. 1982; see Pettegrew et al. 1987b, 1988a, and 1990b for details of the harvesting of brain tissue, perchloric acid extraction, and ^{31}P NMR analyses).

To interpret ^{31}P NMR spectra correctly, the identities of the individual resonance signals must be carefully verified through the use of appropriate biochemical and spectroscopic procedures. The importance of this verification was recently demonstrated for a prominent ^{31}P NMR resonance at 3.84 ppm (3.84δ) in mammalian brain, which was identified as phosphoethanolamine (Pettegrew et al. 1986). The identification was based on hydrogen-1 and ^{31}P NMR findings (including pH titrations) at 4.7 and 14.1 tesla, as well as thin-layer chromatographic analysis. In addition, L-phosphoserine is a significant contributor to the phosphomono-ester (PME) resonance region in mammalian, including human, brain (Pettegrew et al. 1990b).

A representative high-resolution ^{31}P NMR spectrum of a brain per-chloric acid extract is shown in Figure 12–1. The easily identifiable reso-nances and their chemical shifts (δ) include hexose 6-phosphate (H6P, 4.47δ); the PMEs phosphoethanolamine (3.84δ), L-phosphoserine (3.89δ), and phosphocholine (3.33δ); inorganic orthophosphate (Pi, 2.63δ); the phosphodiesters (PDEs) glycerol 3-phosphoethanolamine (GPE, 0.81δ) and glycerol 3-phosphocholine (GPC, −0.13δ); phospho-creatine (PCr, −3.12δ); the nucleotide triphosphates (especially ATP; γ −5.80δ, α −10.92δ, β −21.4δ); the nucleotide diphosphates (especially ADP; β −6.11δ, α −10.61δ); dinucleotides such as nicotinamide adenine dinucleotide phosphate (NADP, −11.37δ); and a complex resonance band centered around −12.89δ that is composed of nucleoside diphos-

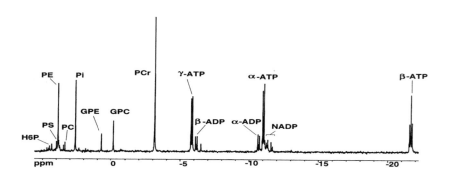

Figure 12–1.   In vitro ^{31}P NMR spectrum at 11.7 tesla resolution of a perchloric acid extract of freeze-clamped brain from a 3-month-old Fischer 344 rat. The readily identifiable resonances and their chemical shifts (δ) include hexose 6-phosphate (H6P, 4.47δ); the phosphomonoesters L-phosphoserine (PS, 3.89δ), phosphoethanolamine (PE, 3.84δ), and phosphocholine (PC, 3.33δ); inorganic orthophosphate (Pi, 2.63δ); the phosphodiesters glycerol 3-phosphoethanolamine (GPE, 0.81δ) and glycerol 3-phosphocholine (GPC, −0.13δ); phosphocreatine (PCr, −3.12δ); the nucleotide triphosphates (especially ATP; γ-ATP, −5.80δ; α-ATP, −10.92δ; β-ATP, −21.45δ); the nucleotide diphosphates (especially ADP; β-ADP, −6.11δ; α-ADP, −10.61δ); dinucleotides such as nicotinamide adenine dinucleotide phosphate (NADP, −11.37δ); and a complex resonance band centered around −12.89δ that is composed of nucleoside diphospho- derivatives such as cytidine diphosphocholine and cytidine diphosphoethanolamine.

pho- derivatives such as uridine diphosphosugars and cytidine diphospho- derivatives such as cytidine diphosphocholine and cytidine diphosphoethanolamine.

The PMEs phosphocholine, phosphoethanolamine, and L-phosphoserine are normally found in abundance in mammalian, including human, brain and are important constituents in the metabolism of their respective phospholipids. The brain concentrations (mM) are phosphoethanolamine $\cong$ 1.5, phosphocholine $\cong$ 0.5, and L-phosphoserine $\cong$ 0.3. The levels of the PMEs are increased approximately threefold in the developing brain during neuritic proliferation (Pettegrew et al. 1990b). Similar high levels of PMEs have been demonstrated in newborn human brain by ^{31}P NMR (Cady et al. 1983). In addition, inositol 1,4,5-triphosphate (Ins(1,4,5)P$_3$) is a PME and is an important second messenger involved in the regulation of intracellular calcium levels (Berridge and Irvine 1984). Ins(1,4,5)P$_3$ is derived from phosphatidylinositol (4,5)-diphosphate [PtdI(4,5)P$_2$], which constitutes approximately 1%–10% of the total PtdI (Majerus et al. 1986). Because the PtdI concentration in mammalian brain is approximately 1.9 mM (McIlwain and Bachelard 1985), the normal concentration of PtdI(4,5)P$_2$ is approximately 0.01–0.1 mM. Therefore, the levels of Ins(1,4,5)P$_3$ normally found in brain tissue would be below the limits of detection by in vivo ^{31}P NMR. The PMEs are produced by 1) phosphorylation of their respective bases by kinases, 2) phospholipase C cleavage of their respective phospholipids, or 3) phosphodiesterase cleavage of their respective PDEs such as GPC and GPE. The PMEs are broken down by phospholipase D to release Pi and the constituent base.

GPC and GPE are also in high abundance in human brain. The PDEs are products of phospholipase A$_1$ + A$_2$ activity and are converted to their respective PMEs by PDE phosphodiesterase activity. In spite of their high abundance in brain, the physiological function of the PDEs remains unknown.

Periods of brain development. Brain maturation and development can be arbitrarily divided into four periods in the rat (McIlwain and Bachelard 1985). Period I is the period of cellular division and extends up to birth. The rat brain at birth has approximately 15% of its adult weight and has no recordable electrical activity. In period II (from birth to 10 days of age), there is growth in the size of individual cells, rapid outgrowth of axons, and rapid development of dendritic connections. There is also a rapid increase in brain lipid content, which peaks at approximately 10 days. In period III (10–20 days of age), synaptic densities and the number of nerve terminals rapidly increase and electroencephalographic activity develops. During this period there are increases in cell volume and the associated K^+ space, with decreases in the extracellular Na^+ and C^- spaces. The rates of glucose uptake, glycolysis, and oxidative phosphorylation all steadily increase from birth to reach their adult levels during period III. Naturally occurring cell death has been demonstrated to occur during the period of synaptogenesis, which would correspond to periods II and III in the rat (Clarke 1985; Cowan et al. 1984; Oppenheim 1985; Pittman and Oppenheim 1979). Adenosine triphosphatase activity, including activity requiring added Na^+ and K^+, increases during periods II and III. Period IV extends from 20 days and is associated with active myelination but little further brain growth. During this period creatine phosphokinase activity reaches maximal levels. Senescence in rats is thought to develop after 12 months of age and certainly by 24 months of age.

Animal studies of brain development and aging.   There are striking effects of animal development and aging on the brain levels of α-GP, phosphoethanolamine, phosphocholine, GPE, GPC, PCr, and Pi (Pettegrew et al. 1990b). The PMEs (α-GP, phosphoethanolamine, and phosphocholine) are high in the immature brain and rapidly decrease from the newborn period to 3 months of age ($P = .0001$). The levels of α-GP and phosphocholine then remain relatively constant until 12 months of age, but the levels of phosphoethanolamine increase slightly ($.01 < P < .05$). From 12 to 24 months, the levels of phosphocholine decrease ($.0001 < P < .001$). In contrast, the PDEs (GPE and GPC) are very low or undetectable in the newborn period and then rise rapidly up to 3 months of age ($P = .0001$), after which the levels rise at a slower rate up to 24 months of age. The PME-to-PDE ratio, which is an estimate of membrane phospholipid anabolic/catabolic activity (Pettegrew et al. 1987b), is high in the newborn period, decreases rapidly up to 3 months of age ($P = .0001$), and then remains relatively constant up to 12 months of age. After 12 months of age, the PME-to-PDE ratio decreases slightly ($.01 < P < .05$), suggesting that membrane phospholipid breakdown is proceeding slightly faster than membrane phospholipid synthesis.

Possible enzymatic causes for the high PME levels during brain development are 1) increased choline, ethanolamine, or serine kinase activity; 2) increased phospholipase C activity; 3) increased glycerophosphodiesterase activity; 4) decreased cytidine diphosphate–choline phosphotransferase activity; 5) decreased PME phosphatase activity; and 6) decreased phospholipase D activity. Possible enzymatic causes for the low PDE levels during brain development are decreased phospholipase A_1 and A_2 activity and decreased glycerophosphodiesterase activity.

These ^{31}P NMR results (Pettegrew et al. 1990b) tentatively suggest very high phospholipid anabolic activity without appreciable catabolic activity from 12 hours to 10 days of age. This would coincide with an increase in the size of neuronal cells, the rapid outgrowth of axons, and the rapid development of dendritic connections reported to occur in period II. After 10 days of age, there is a rapid increase in PDEs, which are catabolic breakdown products of membrane phospholipids. The PME levels start to decrease at 10 days of age, but the PME-to-PDE ratio remains high (> 10). The increasing PDEs observed from 10 to 30 days of age could represent the metabolic correlates of naturally occurring cell death and the remodeling neuritic connections. Cell death has been demonstrated to occur naturally during neural development and, in particular, occurs at about the time of rapid synaptogenesis, which is from birth to 20 days of age in the rat (Clarke 1985; Cowan et al. 1984; Oppenheim 1985; Pittman and Oppenheim 1979). From 1 to 3 months of age, the PMEs continue to decrease and the PDEs continue to increase, although not as rapidly as before. The PME-to-PDE ratio falls from 10 to 2, indicating that the rate of phospholipid synthesis is decreasing. The changes in PME and PDE occurring from 1 to 3 months of age could reflect active myelination, which is known to occur during this time in the rat. After 3 months of age, the turnover rate for phospholipids (PME-to-PDE) remains relatively constant until 12 months of age. From 12 to 24 months of age, the PME-to-PDE ratio decreases further ($.01 < P < .05$), suggesting that membrane catabolism is proceeding slightly faster than anabolism.

PCr is the most metabolically labile of the brain high-energy phosphates. Levels of PCr are quite low in the newborn period and appear to decrease even further up to 5 days of age. After 5 days of age, the PCr levels rapidly increase up to 1 month of age, with less rapid increases between 1 and 3 months of age (12 hours versus 3 months; $P = .0001$). After 3 months of age, the PCr levels undergo less dramatic but steady increases up to 24 months of age. In contrast, the levels of Pi are relatively high in the newborn, with decreases up to 5 days of age followed by increases up to 10 days of age. After 10 days of age, the Pi levels drop rapidly until 3 months of age ($.01 < P < .05$). From 3 months of age until 12 months of age, the Pi levels appear to increase slightly, with more rapid increases from 12 to 24 months of age.

The PCr-to-Pi ratio provides a convenient measure of the energy status of the brain, as it is the ratio of the most labile form of high-energy phosphate (PCr) to the ultimate breakdown product of all high-energy phosphates (Pi). The PCr-to-Pi ratio is quite low in the newborn period until 5 days of age, after which time the PCr-to-Pi ratio increases rapidly up to 3 months of age ($P = .0001$). After 3 months of age, the PCr-to-Pi ratio remains relatively constant up to 24 months of age. The rapid increase in the PCr-to-Pi ratio up to 1 month of age correlates with the development of the glycolytic and oxidative pathways, increasing Na^+-K^+ ATPase activity, and the onset of electroencephalographic activity. The PCr-to-Pi ratio appears to increase slightly after 12 months of age, suggesting decreased utilization of PCr. The brain levels of ATP do not undergo similar changes; there are no significant differences in brain ATP content between animals of 12 hours versus 3 months, 3 months versus 12 months, or 12 months versus 24 months of age.

In Vivo Studies

Brain chemistry also can be assessed in vivo using ^{31}P NMR spectroscopy. [31]P has a nuclear magnetic moment and is present in 100% natural abundance, so no isotope has to be given to the subject. ^{31}P NMR spectroscopy provides a direct in vivo assessment of the brain membrane phospholipid and high-energy phosphate metabolism. The PME and PDE resonances in mammalian brain originate predominantly from the precursors and breakdown products, respectively, of membrane phospholipids (Pettegrew et al. 1986, 1987a). The PCr, ATP, ADP, and Pi levels reflect the state of energy metabolism (Pettegrew et al. 1987a). In addition, the intracellular pH can be directly assessed (Petroff et al. 1985; Pettegrew et al. 1988a). Because NMR spectroscopy is safe and noninvasive, repeated measurements can be carried out in the same individual over a period of time, making longitudinal studies possible.

In vivo ^{31}P NMR spectra on human subjects have been obtained using a Signa system (Medical Systems Operations, General Electric Co., Milwaukee, Wisconsin) with the spectroscopy research accessory. The field strength is 1.5 tesla, yielding a proton frequency of 63.970 MHz and a phosphorus frequency of 25.895 MHz. The subject is placed supine on the NMR magnet transport table, and the head is positioned inside a Plexiglas head holder containing a support bracket for securing a surface coil. The surface coil is positioned over the head to sample signals from the dorsal prefrontal cortex.

All subjects have routine T1-weighted ^{1}H magnetic resonance imaging (MRI) scans in the sagittal, coronal, and axial planes immediately preceding or following the ^{31}P NMR spectroscopy studies. ^{1}H images, which are used to identify the location and volume of brain sampled by spectroscopy, and the ^{31}P NMR spectra, are acquired with the same probe containing an 8-inch ^{31}P surface coil and a 3-inch surface coil dual-tuned at both the ^{31}P and ^{1}H frequencies. ^{1}H images for spectral localization are obtained by transmitting with a Helmholtz body coil and receiving with the 3-inch surface coil. The localized ^{1}H images and the ^{31}P NMR spectra are from approximately 15–20 cm^3 of the dorsal prefrontal cortex (Figure 12–2). The B_0 field is then shimmed on the H_2O ^{1}H signal to a line width of approximately 0.1 ppm.

^{31}P NMR spectra are obtained using a B_1 field gradient and a pulse-acquire sequence. A pulse width of 800 μseconds produces a spectrum with PCr-to-Pi and PME-to-PDE ratios typical of those of mammalian brain. We have previously pointed out the importance of these considerations (Pettegrew et al. 1983a). Other acquisition parameters are as follows: time to pulse repetition (TR) = 2 seconds, sweep width = 2 kHz, receiver filter = 1 kHz, and number of complex data points = 2048. The integrated spectral areas are the same for TR values of 2, 4, and 6 seconds. Therefore, a TR of 2 seconds is used, allowing a greater signal-to-noise ratio for a fixed total acquisition time without signal saturation.

All spectra are processed on a Nicolet data station (Nicolet Magnetics Corp., Fremont, California) with 5 Hz exponential multiplication, first- and second-order phase correction to bring all peaks into absorption mode, and baseline correction by means of a series of linear tilts between known baseline points. Integrated areas are then calculated using the GENCAP program, which fits the spectrum with a series of Lorentzian lines. Known doublets, such as the ionized ends region, are fitted with two Lorentzians, and known triplets, such as the middles region, are fitted with three Lorentzians. The PME and PDE peaks are fitted with one, two, or three Lorentzian lines to obtain the most accurate fit. For each spectrum, the integrated areas of the PME, Pi, PDE, PCr, ionized ends (γ-ATP + β-ADP), esterified ends (α-ATP + α-ADP), and middles (β-ATP) regions are determined. From these integrated areas, the mole percentages of PME, Pi, PDE, PCr, ATP, and ADP are calculated as the integrated area under the resonance peak divided by the total spectral integrated area (Figure 12–3). The intracellular pH is determined by the chemical shift difference between the PCr and Pi peaks (Petroff et al. 1985) or between the γ and α peaks of ATP (Pettegrew et al. 1988a). Our in vivo results

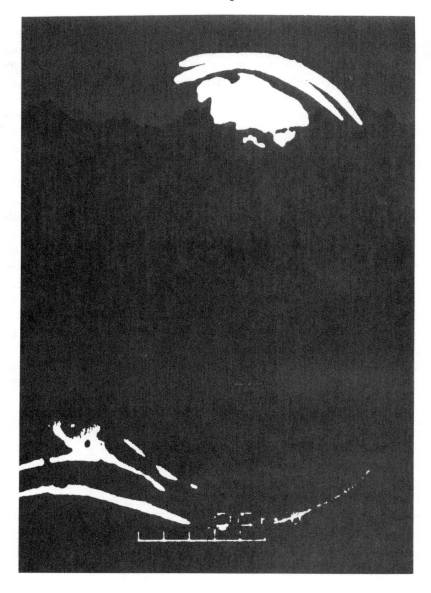

Figure 12–2. ^{1}H sagittal brain image demonstrating the region sampled by the 7.5-cm dual-tuned (^{1}H-^{31}P) surface coil. The sampled region is approximately 15–20 cm^{3} of the dorsal prefrontal cortex. The ^{31}P spectrum of this region is given in Figure 12–3. *Source.* Reprinted from Pettegrew JW, Keshavan MS, Panchalingam K, et al.: "Alterations in Brain High-Energy Phosphate and Membrane Phospholipid Metabolism in First-Episode, Drug-Naive Schizophrenics." *Archives of General Psychiatry* 48:563–568, 1991. Used with permission. Copyright 1991, American Medical Association.

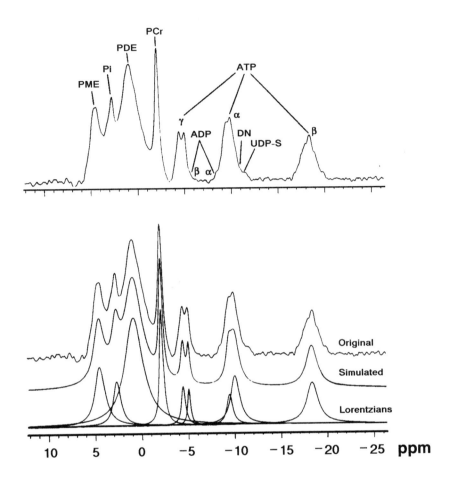

Figure 12–3. In vivo ^{31}P NMR spectra at 1.5 tesla resolution obtained from the dorsal prefrontal cortex after 600 acquisitions. *Top:* Spectrum gives peak assignments for phosphomonoesters (PME); inorganic orthophosphate (Pi); phosphodiesters (PDE); phosphocreatine (PCr); γ, α, and β resonances of ATP; β and α resonances of ADP; dinucleotide phosphates (DN); and uridine diphosphosugars (UDP-S). *Bottom:* Set of three spectra show an original spectrum *(top)*, an original spectrum deconvoluted into component Lorentzian peaks *(bottom)*, and a simulated spectrum obtained by adding the Lorentzian peaks *(center)*. *Source.* Reprinted from Pettegrew JW, Keshavan MS, Panchalingam K, et al.: "Alterations in Brain High-Energy Phosphate and Membrane Phospholipid Metabolism in First-Episode, Drug-Naive Schizophrenics." *Archives of General Psychiatry* 48:563–568, 1991. Used with permission. Copyright 1991, American Medical Association.

compare quite favorably with previously published in vitro results (Cohen et al. 1984; Glonek et al. 1982; Pettegrew et al. 1987a, 1990b), verifying the validity of the in vivo method used in the present study. Test-retest and interrater reliability results give standard deviations of less than 5% of the mean for each parameter ($N = 10$).

Comparison of In Vitro and In Vivo Findings

The PME, Pi, PDE, and PCr resonances of brain are not completely resolved in the unprocessed in vivo ^{31}P NMR spectrum obtained at 1.5 tesla. This is probably due to a combination of at least four factors:

1. The NMR natural line widths for these in vivo brain chemical species are probably broader than those for the same chemical species in solution, indicating longer correlation times (τ_c) for the species in vivo.
2. Some of these chemical species could be in chemical exchange with divalent cations such as Ca^{2+} and Mg^{2+}. If the chemical exchange rate is intermediate with respect to the observed frequency (ω_0), this could lead to line broadening (Pettegrew et al. 1988a). The PME, PDE, and Pi have been shown to chelate di- and trivalent cations in solution (Panchalingam et al. 1987), so this possibility also could exist in vivo.
3. There is decreased chemical shift dispersion at 1.5 tesla compared with B_0 fields of 4.7 tesla or higher.
4. The B_0 field homogeneity across the human head is not as good as that attainable across smaller samples (5- to 20-mm diameters) with better dielectric homogeneity.

Normal Brain Development and Aging

To properly interpret the findings in schizophrenic subjects, it is important to know how high-energy phosphate and membrane phospholipid metabolism change in normal human brain development and aging. In vivo ^{31}P NMR of the dorsal prefrontal cortex was performed on 29 volunteers ages 12–81 years. All subjects had normal medical and neurological examinations, no subject met DSM-III-R (American Psychiatric Association 1987) criteria for any psychiatric disorder, and no subject had a positive family history for neuropsychiatric disorders. There was a significant decrease in the levels of PME ($P = .01$; $r = .52$) and a significant increase in the levels of PDE (P = .01; r = .52) with age. There were no age-related changes in the levels of PCr, Pi, or ATP.

The studies in normal human volunteers show effects of brain development and aging similar to those demonstrated in the Fischer 344 rat (Pettegrew et al. 1990b). The PME increase between the ages of 10 and 20 years remains relatively stable up to 40–50 years and then slowly declines after 50 years of age. The PDE decrease between the ages of 10 and 20 years remains relatively stable up to 40–50 years and then slowly increases after 50 years of age. The changes in brain levels of PME and PDE in individuals between 10 and 20 years of age probably reflect increasing membrane anabolic and decreasing membrane catabolic activity between these ages. The decreasing PME and increasing PDE that occur over age 50 presumably reflect the loss of dendritic spines and processes that occurs with aging.

Schizophrenic Patients and Control Subjects

Brain high-energy phosphate and membrane phospholipid metabolism were investigated under resting conditions in the dorsal prefrontal cortex of neuroleptic-naive, first-episode schizophrenic patients and healthy controls matched for age, sex, race, education, and parental education. Neuroleptic-naive patients were chosen because of the known lasting effects of neuroleptics on membrane phospholipids (Essali et al. 1989). Patients at an early stage of the illness were chosen to exclude the possible effects of length of illness and hospitalization. Eleven schizophrenic patients (7 males, 4 females; 24.4 ± 1.4 years [mean ± SEM]; 7 white, 4 black; 11.7 ± 0.8 years of education) and 10 matched healthy controls (6 males, 4 females; 24.1 ± 1.8 years; 7 white, 2 black, 1 Asian American; 12.7 ± 0.3 years of education) were studied.

Patients were assessed with the Schedule for Affective Disorders and Schizophrenia (SADS) (Endicott and Spitzer 1978) and met both DSM-III-R and Research Diagnostic Criteria (RDC) (Spitzer et al. 1978) for schizophrenia. The DSM-III-R subclassifications for the patients were 6 undifferentiated and 5 paranoid. None had been previously treated with neuroleptics as reported by the patients' families or the referring physicians. The mean illness duration was 19.1 ± 5.9 months. None had a history of persistent substance abuse or met DSM-III-R criteria for it. Physical examination did not reveal abnormalities in any patient. The patients also were assessed using the Brief Psychiatric Rating Scale (BPRS) (Overall and Gorham 1962). All the patients were followed for at least 6 months

after entry into the study to ensure diagnostic stability. The control subjects were selected from among students and hospital staff. Psychiatric,
medical, and family history data were obtained using a structured form.
All patients and control subjects signed informed consent forms.

There were no significant group differences between the patients
and control subjects for age, sex, race, education, or parental education.
The MRI results were normal in the schizophrenic patients and control
subjects as reported by experienced neuroradiologists. The following
metabolic alterations were observed in the dorsal prefrontal cortex of the
schizophrenic patients:

- Decreased levels of PME (schizophrenic patients = 15.5 ± 0.9, control subjects = 20.3 ± 0.9; $P = .002$)
- Increased levels of PDE (schizophrenic patients = 36.4 ± 1.5, control
  subjects = 32.2 ± 0.6; $P = .02$)
- Increased levels of ATP (schizophrenic patients = 9.6 ± 0.5, control
  subjects = 7.4 ± 0.4; $P = .02$)
- Decreased levels of Pi (schizophrenic patients = 7.9 ± 0.5, control
  subjects = 9.9 ± 0.5; $P = .01$)

There were no group differences in the levels of PCr, ADP, or intracellular pH.

Possible causes for decreased observable levels of PME in schizophrenic brain are decreased kinase activity, decreased phospholipase C
activity, decreased PDE phosphodiesterase activity, increased phospholipase D activity, increased chemical exchange with divalent cations
leading to decreased NMR observability, and increased τ_c with resulting
decreased NMR observability. Possible causes for increased PDE in schizophrenic brain include decreased PDE phosphodiesterase activity and
increased phospholipase $A_1 + A_2$ activity. Gattaz et al. (1987) reported increased activity of phospholipase A_2 in schizophrenia. Other possible
causes of the increased observable PDE are decreased τ_c with increased
NMR observability or decreased chemical exchange with divalent cations
resulting in increased NMR observability. Decreased PDE phosphodiesterase activity could account for both the decreased PME and the
increased PDE levels observed in the schizophrenic patients studied.

Our findings of decreased PME and increased PDE levels also could
suggest decreased synthesis and increased breakdown of membrane
phospholipids in schizophrenia. Similar results are observed in normal
aging in animals by in vitro ^{31}P NMR (Cady et al. 1983) and humans by in

vivo ^{31}P NMR spectroscopy (Pettegrew et al. 1990a). Demisch et al. (1987) reported a significantly decreased incorporation of ^{14}C-labeled arachidonic acid in PtdC, PtdE, and PtdI in patients with schizoaffective and schizophreniform disorders, which could suggest decreased membrane phospholipid synthesis. Decreased levels of membrane PtdC have been observed in erythrocytes in some schizophrenic patients (Henn 1980; Hitzemann et al. 1984; Stevens 1972). All the schizophrenic patients in the present study had normal MRI findings (as reported by neuroradiologists) at the time of their ^{31}P NMR studies. It is possible, therefore, that the PME and PDE alterations could represent metabolic alterations that antedate the onset of anatomical changes.

The increased ATP and decreased Pi observed in the present study suggest decreased ATP utilization with decreased production of Pi. These findings are consistent with hypoactivity of the dorsal prefrontal cortex as suggested by decreased cerebral blood flow and decreased uptake of 2-deoxyglucose (Buchsbaum et al. 1982; Ingvar and Franzen 1974; Weinberger et al. 1986). Both cerebral blood flow and 2-deoxyglucose uptake are indirect measures of cerebral energy metabolism. The uptake of glucose and presumably 2-deoxyglucose are dependent upon normal membrane properties (Carruthers et al. 1989), and the decreased uptake of 2-deoxyglucose observed in some schizophrenic patients also could reflect altered membrane phospholipids.

Schizophrenic Patients and Autistic Patients

Adult autistic patients of normal IQ who were similar in age to the schizophrenic patients and share some of the negative symptoms were studied by in vivo ^{31}P NMR spectroscopy using the identical protocol used for the schizophrenic patients (Minshew et al. 1990, 1991, in press; Pettegrew et al. 1989). These autistic patients did not have altered levels of brain PME or PDE. However, they had decreased levels of ATP, which is the opposite of what was observed in the schizophrenic patients. The decreased levels of ATP suggest increased ATP utilization in the autistic patients. This is consistent with a positron-emission tomography (PET) study of 12 young adult autistic men, which reported an increase in metabolic rate for glucose in hippocampus, thalamus, basal ganglia, and frontal, parietal, temporal, and occipital cortices (Rumsey et al. 1985).

Implications

Schizophrenia, Normal Aging, and Alzheimer's Disease

It is of interest that the changes in PME and PDE observed in schizophrenic patients are distinct and in the opposite direction from those observed with Alzheimer's disease, which is associated with increases in brain PME early in the course of the disease. Elevated brain levels of PDE occur later in the course of Alzheimer's disease and probably reflect the onset of membrane degenerative changes (Brown et al. 1989; Pettegrew et al. 1984, 1987a, 1988b, 1988c, 1990b).

As previously mentioned, the changes observed in schizophrenia are quite similar to those observed in normal aging in which the brain levels of PME are decreased and PDE are increased (Pettegrew et al. 1987a). From this perspective, schizophrenia could be considered a form of premature brain aging, perhaps involving only certain neural systems. This formulation would be in keeping with the concept of dementia praecox put forth by Kraepelin (1919/1971) and Morel (1860). The normal MRI findings reported for all the schizophrenic patients in our study suggest that the PME and PDE alterations could represent metabolic alterations that antedate the onset of anatomical changes. This could provide a possible metabolic explanation for the development of cerebral atrophy observed in some schizophrenic patients (Andreasen 1988; Andreasen et al. 1986), including the affected twin of monozygotic twins discordant for schizophrenia (Suddath et al. 1990).

Schizophrenia and Programmed Synaptic Pruning

The findings of decreased PME and increased PDE in first-episode, drug-naive schizophrenic patients also could be due to abnormal brain development (Feinberg 1982; Weinberger 1987). There is now substantial evidence for programmed neuronal cell loss, loss of callosal axons, and synaptic elimination in normal brain development in animals and humans (Cowan et al. 1984; Huttenlocher 1979; Huttenlocher et al. 1982; Purves and Lichtman 1980; Rakic and Riley 1983).

Our in vivo ^{31}P NMR study indicated that the cell bodies, processes, and terminals in the sampled area of the dorsal prefrontal cortex of the schizophrenic patients contained depressed levels of PME and elevated levels of PDE as compared with the control subjects. In vivo ^{31}P NMR studies of healthy volunteers between ages 12 and 85 years also revealed a transient decrease in the levels of PME and an increase in the levels of PDE during adolescence (10–20 years) (Panchalingam et al. 1990). However, the decreased PME and increased PDE levels observed in the schizophrenic patients appeared to be more pronounced than in the healthy volunteers of comparable age. This suggests decreased synthesis and enhanced breakdown of membranes in the schizophrenic patients, which could be due to altered timing or abnormal enhancement of normal programmed synaptic pruning during adolescence as initially suggested by Feinberg (1982) and demonstrated to occur in the prefrontal cortex of humans during adolescence by Huttenlocher (1979). An exaggeration of these regressive synaptic events involving apical and basal dendrites could produce brain structural changes similar to those observed in schizophrenia in which the predominant reduction is in gray but not white matter. An exaggeration of normal neuronal cell death should produce decreased numbers of neurons and their projection axons and, therefore, reduce the volume of both gray and white matter.

Schizophrenia and Prefrontal Glutamatergic Pathways

The descending prefrontal glutamatergic pathway is a major input to both the striatum and the limbic cortex. Exaggerated synaptic pruning of prefrontal-limbic glutamatergic axonal terminals could produce a reduced neuropil volume, resulting in what might appear as an enhanced clustering of cells as observed for pre–α-cells in the parahippocampal gyrus (Falkai et al. 1988). Excessive pruning of prefrontal-striatal glutamatergic axonal terminals ending on striatal dopaminergic terminals could decrease the tonic release of dopamine from the dopaminergic terminals, resulting in secondary upregulation of the postsynaptic dopaminergic receptors.

A number of postmortem studies have demonstrated increased numbers of D_2 receptors in the caudate and putamen of patients with schizophrenia (Jaskiw and Kleinman 1988; Seeman et al. 1984), but a study by Kornhuber et al. (1989) suggests that this is secondary to neuroleptic treatment within 3 months of death. Wong et al. (1986) reported increased numbers of D_2 receptors in the striatum of drug-naive schizophrenic patients in an in vivo PET study, but this finding was not replicated (Farde et al. 1987).

The phasic release of dopamine is thought to be responsive to stress. With upregulation of postsynaptic dopaminergic receptors, stress could cause exaggerated mesolimbic activity resulting in positive symptoms. Neuroleptics that block postsynaptic D_2 receptors could modulate the mesolimbic activity back toward normal. This formulation was suggested by Grace (1991).

Potential Therapeutic Effect of Neurotrophic Agents

Premature aging of the prefrontal cortex or an exaggeration or altered timing of the normal synaptic pruning of the prefrontal cortex, which occurs in adolescence, could potentially produce the PME and PDE findings observed in the schizophrenic patients in our study. Should decreased brain PME and increased PDE be found in a much larger sample of schizophrenic patients, then consideration should be given to the possible use of brain trophic factors early in the course of schizophrenia. The goal would be to identify by ^{31}P NMR those individuals who demonstrate the PME and PDE changes early in the course of the illness or, even better, prior to the onset of symptoms. These individuals would then be candidates for neurotrophic therapy to slow, stop, or even reverse the membrane alterations. This is obviously highly speculative, and even if this approach should prove beneficial, it is still far into the future. However, by starting to plan for the future now, perhaps we can make the future less far off.

The ability of ^{31}P NMR to monitor high-energy phosphates as well as membrane phospholipid metabolites could provide new insights not previously available with other techniques. ^{31}P NMR spectroscopy also appears to be a practicable procedure for longitudinal studies, which can potentially provide new information on the possible evolution of regional biochemical changes in schizophrenia.

References

Ackerman JH, Grove TH, Wong GG, et al: Mapping of metabolites in whole animals by ^{31}P NMR using surface coils. Nature 283:167–170, 1980

American Psychiatric Association: Diagnostic and Statistical Manual of Mental Disorders, Third Edition, Revised. Washington, DC, American Psychiatric Association, 1987

Andreasen NC: Brain imaging: applications in psychiatry. Science 239:1381–1388, 1988

Andreasen N, Nasrallah HA, Dunn V, et al: Structural abnormalities in the frontal system in schizophrenia. Arch Gen Psychiatry 43:136–144, 1986

Barany M, Glonek T: Identification of diseased states by phosphorus-31 NMR, in Phosphorus-31 NMR, Principles and Applications. Edited by Gorenstein DG. New York, Academic Press, 1984, pp 511–515

Berman KF, Illowsky BP, Weinberger DR: Physiological dysfunction of dorsolateral prefrontal cortex in schizophrenia. Arch Gen Psychiatry 45:616–622, 1988

Berridge MJ, Irvine RF: Inositol triphosphate, a novel second messenger in cellular signal transduction. Nature 312:315–321, 1984

Blass JP, Hanin I, Barclay L, et al: Red blood cell abnormalities in Alzheimer disease. J Am Geriatr Soc 33:401–405, 1985

Brown GG, Levine SR, Gorell JM, et al: In vivo ^{31}P NMR profiles of Alzheimer's disease and multiple subcortical infarct dementia. Neurology 39:1423–1427, 1989

Buchsbaum MS: Position emission tomography in schizophrenia, in Psychopharmacology: The Third Generation of Progress. Edited by Meltzer HY. New York, Raven, 1987, pp 783–792

Buchsbaum MS, Ingvar DH, Kessler R, et al: Cerebral glucography with positron tomography. Arch Gen Psychiatry 39:251–259, 1982

Butterfield DA, Markesbery WR: Specificity of biophysical and biochemical alterations in erythrocyte membranes with neurological disorders. J Neurol Sci 97:261–271, 1980

Butterfield DA, Oeswein JW, Markesbery WR: Electron spin resonance study of membrane protein alterations in erythrocytes in Huntington's disease (letter). Nature 267:453–455, 1977

Butterfield DA, Oeswein JW, Prunty ME, et al: Increased sodium plus potassium adenosine triphosphatase activity in erythrocyte membranes in Huntington's disease. Ann Neurol 4:60–62, 1978

Butterfield DA, Nicholas MM, Markesbery WR: Evidence for an increased rate of choline efflux across erythrocyte membranes in Alzheimer's disease. Neurochem Res 10:909–918, 1985

Cady E, Dawson M, Hope P, et al: Non-invasive investigations of cerebral metabolism in newborn infants by phosphorus nuclear magnetic resonance spectroscopy. Lancet 1:1059–1062, 1983

Carruthers A, Helgerson AL, Herbert DN, et al: Effects of calcium ATP and lipids on human erythrocyte sugar transport. Ann N Y Acad Sci 568:52–67, 1989

Chance B, Nakase Y, Bond M, et al: Detection of ^{31}P nuclear magnetic resonance signals in brain by in vivo and freeze trapped assays. Proc Natl Acad Sci U S A 75:4925–4929, 1978

Clarke PG: Neuronal death in the development of the vertebrate nervous system. Trends Neurosci 8:345–349, 1985

Cohen MM, Pettegrew JW, Kopp SJ, et al: P-31 nuclear magnetic resonance analysis of brain: normoxic and anoxic brain slices. Neurochem Res 9(6):785–801, 1984

Cowan WM, Fawcett JW, O'Leary DD, et al: Regressive events in neurogenesis. Science 225:1258–1265, 1984

Demisch L, Gerbaldo H, Heinz K, et al: Transmembranal signalling in schizophrenic and affective disorders: studies on arachidonic acid and phospholipids. Schizophr Res 22:275–282, 1987

Diamond JM, Matsuyama SS, Meier K, et al: Elevation of erythrocyte countertransport rates in Alzheimer's dementia (letter). N Engl J Med 309:1061–1062, 1983

Endicott J, Spitzer RL: A diagnostic interview: the Schedule for Affective Disorders and Schizophrenia. Arch Gen Psychiatry 35:837–844, 1978

Essali MA, Das I, deBelleroche J, et al: The platelet polyphosphoinositide system in schizophrenia: pathological and pharmacological implications (abstract). Schizophr Res 2:148, 1989

Falkai P, Bogerts B, Rozumek M: Cell loss and volume reduction in the entorhinal cortex of schizophrenics. European Archives of Psychiatry and Neurological Sciences 24:515–521, 1988

Farde L, Wiesel FA, Hall H, et al: No D2 receptor increase in PET study of schizophrenia (letter). Arch Gen Psychiatry 44:671–672, 1987

Feinberg I: Schizophrenia: caused by a fault in programmed synaptic elimination during adolescence? J Psychiatr Res 17(4):319–334, 1982

Gattaz W, Kolisch M, Thuren T, et al: Increased plasma phospholipase A2 activity in schizophrenic patients: reduction after neuroleptic therapy. Biol Psychiatry 22:421–426, 1987

Glonek T, Kopp SJ, Kot E, et al: P-31 nuclear magnetic resonance analysis of brain: the perchloric acid extract spectrum. J Neurochem 39:1210–1219, 1982

Grace AA: Phasic versus tonic dopamine release and the modulation of dopamine system responsivity: a hypothesis for the etiology of schizophrenia. Neuroscience 41:1–24, 1991

Heaton R: Wisconsin Card Sorting Test. Odessa, TX, Psychological Assessment Resources, 1985

Henn F: Biological concepts in schizophrenia research, in Perspectives in Schizophrenia Research. Edited by Baxter C, Melnachuk T. New York, Raven, 1980, p 209–223

Hitzemann R, Hirschowitz D, Garver D: Membrane abnormalities in the psychoses and affective disorders. J Psychiatr Res 18:319–326, 1984

Huttenlocher PR: Synaptic density in human frontal cortex: developmental changes and effects of aging. Brain Res 163:195–205, 1979

Huttenlocher PR, deCourten C, Garey LJ, et al: Synaptogenesis in human visual cortex—evidence for synapse elimination during normal development. Neurosci Lett 33:247–252, 1982

Ingvar DH, Franzen G: Abnormalities of cerebral blood flow distribution in patients with chronic schizophrenia. Acta Psychiatr Scand 50:425–462, 1974

Jaskiw G, Kleinman J: Postmortem neurochemistry studies in schizophrenia, in Schizophrenia: A Scientific Focus. Edited by Schulz SC, Tamminga CA. New York, Oxford University Press, 1988, pp 264–273

Kaiya H, Takeuchi K, Namba M, et al: Abnormal phosphatidylinositol-cycle of platelet membrane in schizophrenia: a preliminary study. Folia Psychiatrica et Neurologica Japonica 38:437–444, 1984

Kornhuber J, Riederer P, Reynolds GP, et al: 3H-spiperone binding sites in postmortem brains from schizophrenic patients: relationship to neuroleptic drug treatment, abnormal movements, and positive symptoms. Journal of Neural Transmission 75:1–10, 1989

Kraepelin E: Dementia Praecox and Paraphrenia (1919). Edinburgh, Churchill Livingstone. Translated by Barclay RM, Robertson GM. New York, R E Krieger, 1971

Majerus PW, Connolly TM, Deckmyn H, et al: The metabolism of phosphoinositide-derived messenger molecules. Science 234:1519–1526, 1986

Maris JM, Evans AE, McLaughlin AC, et al: [31]P nuclear magnetic resonance in situ. N Engl J Med 312:1500–1505, 1985

Markesbery WR, Leung PK, Butterfield DA: Spin label and biochemical studies of erythrocyte membranes in Alzheimer's disease. J Neurol Sci 45:323–330, 1980

McIlwain H, Bachelard HS: Biochemistry and the Central Nervous System. Edinburgh, Churchill Livingstone, 1985, p 291

Miller BL, Jenden D, Tang C, et al: Choline and choline-bound phospholipids in aging and Alzheimer's disease (abstract). Neurology 39 (suppl 1):254, 1989

Minshew NJ, Pettegrew JW, Panchalingam K: Membrane phospholipid alterations observed in Alzheimer's disease are not present in Down's syndrome (abstract). Biol Psychiatry 27(9A):123A–124A, 1990

Minshew NJ, Pettegrew JW, Panchalingam K, et al: Membrane phospholipid and energy metabolism in Down's syndrome are different than in Alzheimer's disease (abstract). Neurology 41 (suppl 1):117, 1991

Minshew NJ, Goldstein G, Dombrowski SM, et al: A preliminary ^{31}P MRS study of autism: evidence for undersynthesis and increased degradation of brain membranes. Biol Psychiatry (in press)

Morel BA: Traitement des Maladies Mentales. Paris, Victor Masson, 1860

Oppenheim RW: Naturally occurring cell death during neural development. Trends Neurosci 8:487–493, 1985

Overall JE, Gorham DR: The Brief Psychiatric Rating Scale. Psychol Rep 10:799–812, 1962

Panchalingam K, Post JFM, Pettegrew JW: Evidence for increased aluminum binding ligands in Alzheimer's disease: a ^{31}P NMR study. Neurology 37 (suppl 1):331, 1987

Panchalingam K, Pettegrew JW, Strychor S, et al: Effect of normal aging on membrane phospholipid metabolism by ^{31}P NMR spectroscopy (abstract). Society for Neuroscience Abstracts 16:843, 1990

Petroff OAC, Pritchard JW, Behar KL, et al: Cerebral intracellular pH by ^{31}P nuclear magnetic resonance spectroscopy. Neurology 35:781–788, 1985

Pettegrew JW, Nichols JS, Stewart RM: Fluorescence spectroscopy on Huntington's fibroblasts. J Neurochem 33:905–911, 1979a

Pettegrew JW, Glonek T, Baskin F, et al: Phosphorus-31 NMR of neuroblastoma clonal lines: effect of cell confluency state and dibutyryl cyclic AMP. Neurochem Res 4:795–801, 1979b

Pettegrew JW, Nichols JS, Stewart RM: Studies of fluorescence of fibroblasts from Huntington's disease: evidence of a membrane abnormality (letter). N Engl J Med 300:678, 1979c

Pettegrew JW, Nichols JS, Stewart RM: Membrane studies in Huntington's disease: steady-state and time-dependent fluorescence spectroscopy of intact lymphocytes. J Neurochem 36:1966–1976, 1981

Pettegrew JW, Nichols JS, Minshew NJ, et al: Membrane biophysical studies of lymphocytes and erythrocytes in manic-depressive illness. J Affect Disord 4:237–247, 1982

Pettegrew JW, Minshew NJ, Diehl J, et al: Anatomical considerations for interpreting topical ^{31}P-NMR (letter). Lancet 2:913, 1983a

Pettegrew JW, Minshew NJ, Stewart RM: Dynamic membrane studies in individuals at risk for Huntington's disease. Life Sci 32:1207–1212, 1983b

Pettegrew JW, Minshew NJ, Cohen MM, et al: ^{31}P NMR changes in Alzheimer's and Huntington's disease brain (abstract). Neurology (Minneap) 34 (suppl 1):281, 1984

Pettegrew JW, Kopp SJ, Dadok J, et al: Chemical characterization of a prominent phosphomonoester resonance from mammalian brain: ^{31}P and ^{1}H NMR analysis at 4.7 and 14.1 tesla. Journal of Magnetic Resonance 67:443–450, 1986

Pettegrew JW, Moossy J, Withers G, et al: ^{31}P nuclear magnetic resonance (NMR) spectroscopy of brain aging and Alzheimer's disease. Journal of Neural Transmission 24:261–268, 1987a

Pettegrew JW, Kopp SJ, Minshew NJ, et al: 31P nuclear magnetic resonance studies of phosphoglyceride metabolism in developing and degenerating brain: preliminary observations. J Neuropathol Exp Neurol 46:419–430, 1987b

Pettegrew JW, Withers G, Panchalingam K, et al: Considerations for brain pH assessment by ^{31}P NMR. Magn Reson Imaging 6:135–142, 1988a

Pettegrew JW, Panchalingam K, Moossy J, et al: Correlation of phosphorus-31 magnetic resonance spectroscopy and morphological findings in Alzheimer's disease. Arch Neurol 45:1093–1096, 1988b

Pettegrew JW, Moossy J, Withers G, et al: ^{31}P NMR nuclear magnetic resonance study of the brain in Alzheimer's disease. J Neuropathol Exp Neurol 47:3, 235–248, 1988c

Pettegrew JW, Minshew NJ, Payton JB: ^{31}P NMR in normal IQ adult autistics (abstract). Biol Psychiatry 25:182A–183A, 1989

Pettegrew JW, Panchalingam K, Strychor S, et al: Analysis of membrane phospholipids in Alzheimer's disease brain by ^{31}P NMR (abstract). Society for Neuroscience Abstracts 16:498, 1990a

Pettegrew JW, Panchalingam K, Withers G, et al: Changes in brain energy and phospholipid metabolism during development and aging in the Fischer 344 rat. J Neuropathol Exp Neurol 49:237–249, 1990b

Pittman R, Oppenheim RW: Cell death of motoneurons in the chick embryo spinal cord, IV: evidence that a functional neuromuscular interaction is involved in the regulation of naturally occurring cell death and the stabilization of synapses. J Comp Neurol 187:425–446, 1979

Purves D, Lichtman JW: Elimination of synapses in the developing nervous system. Science 210:153–157, 1980

Rakic P, Riley KP: Overproduction and elimination of retinal axons in the fetal rhesus monkey. Science 219:1441–1444, 1983

Rotrosen J, Wolkin A: Phospholipid and prostaglandin hypothesis in schizophrenia, in Psychopharmacology: The Third Generation of Progress. Edited by Meltzer HY. New York, Raven, 1987, pp 759–764

Rumsey JM, Duara R, Grady C, et al: Brain metabolism in autism: resting cerebral glucose utilization rates as measured with positron emission tomography. Arch Gen Psychiatry 42:448–455, 1985

Seeman P, Ulpian C, Bergeron C, et al: Bimodal distribution of dopamine receptor densities in brains of schizophrenics. Science 225:728–731, 1984

Sherman KA, Gibson GE, Blass JP: Human red blood cell choline uptake with age and Alzheimer's disease. Neurobiol Aging 7:205–209, 1986

Spitzer RL, Endicott J, Robins E: Research Diagnostic Criteria (RDC) for a Selected Group of Function Disorders, 3rd Edition. New York, New York State Psychiatric Institute, 1978

Stevens JD: The distribution of phospholipid fractions in the red cell membrane of schizophrenics. Schizophr Bull 6:60–61, 1972

Suddath RL, Christison GW, Torrey EF, et al: Anatomical abnormalities in the brains of monozygotic twins discordant for schizophrenia. N Engl J Med 322:789–794, 1990

Weinberger DR: Implications of normal brain development for the pathogenesis of schizophrenia. Arch Gen Psychiatry 44:660–669, 1987

Weinberger DR, Berman KF, Zec RF: Psychologic dysfunction of the dorsolateral prefrontal cortex in schizophrenia. Arch Gen Psychiatry 43:114–124, 1986

Wong DF, Wagner HN Jr, Tune LE, et al: Positron emission tomography reveals elevated D2 dopamine receptors in drug-naive schizophrenics. Science 234:1558–1563, 1986 [see Science 235:623, 1987 for erratum]

Zubenko GS, Cohen BM, Reynolds CF, et al: Platelet membrane fluidity in Alzheimer's disease and major depression. Am J Psychiatry 144:860–868, 1987

Chapter 13

Molecular Genetic Research in Schizophrenia

Raymond R. Crowe, M.D.

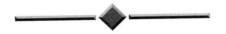

The past decade has witnessed a revolution in medical genetics, with an increasing number of diseases mapped to their respective chromosomes, the responsible genes cloned, and the mutations identified (Martin 1987; White and Caskey 1988). Hopes have been high that these methods, which have worked so well elsewhere in medical genetics, may lead us to the causes of psychiatric diseases (Pardes et al. 1989). The most promising genetic strategy for the study of schizophrenia is linkage analysis. In this chapter I present the principles of linkage analysis and some problems encountered in its use. After summarizing the literature on linkage analysis in schizophrenia, I discuss the results of our research group's Iowa Multiplex Family Study as they relate to linkage.

Linkage Analysis

Linkage analysis is based on the principle that if a disease is caused by a defective gene, its genetic locus can be identified and mapped by ex-

Supported by NIMH Grants R01MH43212 and K01MH00735 (R.R.C.) and R01 MH31593 (Dr. Nancy Andreasen).

amining cotransmission of the disease in multiply affected families with a set of mapped genetic markers (Suarez and Cox 1985). Then, using a variety of molecular genetic techniques, the region of interest can be narrowed until candidate genes are identified and cloned. The ultimate hope is that one of these candidates will prove to be a susceptibility gene for schizophrenia and provide clues to its pathophysiology.

An excellent example of this approach is provided by cystic fibrosis (CF). In 1985 linkage was found to a CF locus on chromosome 7 by three laboratories (Tsui et al. 1985; Wainwright et al. 1985; White et al. 1985). Four years later the responsible gene had been cloned, and over the ensuing years a number of CF-causing mutations to the gene have been pinpointed (Kerem et al. 1989; Riordan et al. 1989; Rommens et al. 1989). Work is now progressing rapidly on the function of the gene, which appears to be involved in transmembrane chloride conductance (Anderson et al. 1991). These advances have revolutionized diagnosis and genetic counseling of CF, and it is hoped that they will ultimately lead to improved treatments as well.

In principle, linkage analysis is straightforward. If a disease is caused by a mutation in a gene, and a genetic marker polymorphism occurs at a nearby locus, then the disease will cosegregate with one of the alleles at the marker locus within families. The farther apart the two loci, the greater the chance of recombination during meiosis. Therefore, the proportion of recombinants and nonrecombinants provides evidence for or against linkage and, second, a measure of the genetic distance between the marker and disease loci. To make the analysis practical, a statistic is needed to analyze across families and measure the degree of cosegregation between loci. The conventional statistic is the lod score, which represents the logarithm of the ratio of the probability of the pedigree assuming a given recombination rate divided by the probability assuming random recombination (the null hypothesis).

In practice, lod scores are calculated over a range of recombination fractions from zero to 50% recombination. Linkage is indicated by a positive lod score, and the genetic distance by the recombination fraction at which the lod score maximizes. Conversely, negative lod scores favor the null hypothesis of nonlinkage. The conventional criterion levels for significance are +3.0 for linkage and −2.0 for the exclusion of linkage. The lod score therefore provides a measure of the degree of confidence with which linkage is supported as well as an estimate of the genetic distance between the marker and the trait loci. Conversely, in the event that linkage does not exist, the lod score provides a measure of the genetic distance over which a gene for the trait can be excluded. It is common to test for linkage over a series of linked marker loci forming a genetic map. In this way, lod scores can be calculated over extensive portions of the chromosomes. It is feasible then, to exclude linkage to a given disease over an entire chromosome.

Although linkage may be straightforward in principle, it can be far from it in practice, especially when applied to diseases with complex patterns of inheritance. No disease exemplifies the problems better than schizophrenia (Risch 1990). Linkage (or more correctly, the lod score) assumes that the pedigrees can be dichotomized into affected and unaffected phenotypes. Yet, despite an abundance of data from family, twin, and adoption studies, there is still no consensus on what the affected phenotype should be. It is clear that schizophrenia is inherited and that a spectrum of milder conditions are found among relatives as well. This presents a problem for linkage analysis because the familial rate of schizophrenia is low enough that if the analysis is limited to that diagnosis, only an extensive set of pedigrees would have the necessary statistical power to detect linkage. On the other hand, if the definition of the affected phenotype is broadened to increase power, and some disorders are incorrectly included, the statistical power will be eroded by the creation of false "recombinants." The compromise that is often employed is to perform multiple analyses and include a range of definitions of the affected phenotype. However, this raises the problem of multiple analyses inflating the lod score, about which more will be said later.

A second assumption made in linkage analysis is that the genetic mechanism by which the trait is inherited is known. To compute the lod score, one must know whether the disease is autosomal or sex linked, dominant or recessive. Further, the disease allele frequency must be specified, and incomplete penetrance (e.g., age, sex, or cohort effects) must be modeled. In the event of genetic heterogeneity, the method of pedigree selection can bias the sample toward a particular mode of inheritance. For example, extended pedigrees will select for autosomal dominant while multiplex sibships will select for autosomal recessive inheritance. Because population allele frequencies vary across ethnic groups, the population from which the pedigrees are selected could bias toward a particular disease allele. These uncertainties can make comparisons across studies and pooling of data treacherous.

Another genetic parameter that must be specified in the linkage analysis but that may not be known is penetrance. Unknown penetrance is often circumvented by testing a range of penetrances, but this again introduces the problem of multiple analyses.

A number of the genetic parameters—mode of inheritance, allele frequency, and penetrance—can be estimated from the pedigrees provided they have been ascertained and extended in a systematic manner. However, even this solution is not totally satisfactory because, in the face of genetic heterogeneity, the parameters estimated will represent a mixture of the different genetic forms of the illness and may not be appropriate to any one.

Another challenge to linkage studies of schizophrenia is knowing where to look for linkage among the 3 billion base pairs of DNA that constitute the human genome. Four strategies can be considered. First, a linkage map can be used for a systematic search of the genome. Second, markers yielding positive lod scores for linkage from earlier studies identify regions of interest. Third, candidate genes such as the dopamine receptors can be tested for linkage. Finally, cytogenetic abnormalities associated with the disease may provide a clue to the location of a gene.

Literature Review

It was a cytogenetic clue that first suggested a gene for schizophrenia on chromosome 5 (Bassett et al. 1988; McGillivray et al. 1990). A young, Asian, schizophrenic male was noted to have dysmorphic facial features and a family history consisting of a maternal uncle with a psychotic illness and dysmorphic features similar to those of the patient. The facial dysmorphism prompted a karyotype of the patient, which revealed an inverted duplication of chromosome 5q11-q13 inserted into chromosome 1. His physically and psychiatrically normal mother carried a balanced translocation, but her schizophrenic brother carried the unbalanced duplication found in the patient. Both family members who were trisomic for chromosome 5q11-q13 had schizophrenic symptoms, raising the possibility of a gene predisposing to schizophrenia in this region of chromosome 5.

These two reports highlighted chromosome 5q11-q13 as a region of interest for linkage studies, and fortunately several DNA probes mapping to this region were available. Sherrington et al. (1988) reported strong evidence of linkage between schizophrenia and two DNA probes in this region. Seven multiplex pedigrees were studied, five from Iceland and two from England. The genetic model assumed a disease allele frequency of 0.0085 and autosomal dominant inheritance with incomplete pene-

trance. Three definitions of the affected phenotype were used: schizophrenia; schizophrenia plus schizoid personality, with or without
schizotypal features; and all psychiatric diagnoses. For each phenotypic
classification, linkage analyses were carried out varying the penetrance
from 0.50 to 1.00 in increments of 0.10, and the model that maximized
the lod score was taken as the best-fitting model. An additional analysis
set penetrance near zero, forcing the lod score to be based only on affected subjects and thus free of assumptions about penetrance.

A multipoint analysis for linkage between schizophrenia and two
DNA markers (D5S76 and D5S39) resulted in a lod score of 3.22 when
schizophrenia was taken as the affected phenotype, 4.33 when schizoid
personality was added, and 6.49 when all psychiatric diagnoses were
added. The penetrance-free model did not achieve the nominally significant lod score of 3.0, but it did exceed 2.0, indicating that the findings
were robust to the assumptions of the genetic models used.

Since the Sherrington et al. (1988) report, a number of other investigators have attempted to replicate the finding without success. Kennedy
et al. (1988) studied five DNA loci spanning the chromosome 5q11-q13
region, including the linked markers from the Sherrington et al. (1988)
study, in five branches of an extended North Swedish kindred of schizophrenia. Because this kindred presented few diagnoses other than schizophrenia, that diagnosis comprised the sole affected phenotype. The
genetic model assumed autosomal dominant transmission of a disease
allele with frequency of 0.02 and penetrance of 0.72. Multipoint linkage
analyses excluded the entire region of chromosome 5q11-q13 by virtue of
lod scores lower than −2.0.

Another unsuccessful attempt to replicate the finding was reported
by St. Clair et al. (1989) in 15 multiplex pedigrees from Scotland. One
unusual feature of these pedigrees was the high incidence of bipolar illness: 5 cases of bipolar I disorder and 5 of bipolar II disorder in 7 of the
15 pedigrees. The genetic model assumed autosomal dominant transmission of a disease allele with a frequency of 0.0085 and penetrance of 0.66,
0.77, or 0.94, depending on the affected phenotype. The three respective
phenotypes were schizophrenia, schizoaffective, bipolar, and other functional psychosis; these disorders plus major depressive disorder; and all
psychiatric diagnoses. The DNA probes from the Sherrington et al.
(1988) study were used in multipoint analyses, and the region was excluded by all analyses. All three models excluded the region supporting
linkage in the Sherrington et al. (1988) study. Because the pedigrees contained a high rate of bipolar illness, 6 pedigrees without bipolar disorder

were analyzed separately under the first definition of affected phenotype for linkage to D5S76, the more informative marker in this study. This analysis likewise gave negative lod scores, indicating that the exclusion by the three other analyses was not a function of including bipolar illness in the schizophrenia spectrum.

Detera-Wadleigh et al. (1990) examined the same markers in five North American pedigrees, four of which contributed to the total lod score. The genetic model assumed autosomal dominance with a gene frequency of 0.015 and penetrance of 0.95. The definitions of the affected phenotype were 1) schizophrenic disorder and schizoaffective disorder; 2) those diagnoses plus schizotypal, paranoid, or schizoid personality disorder; and 3) all of those in the first two definitions plus unipolar and bipolar affective disorder. Under the last two models the critical region of chromosome 5 was excluded in a multipoint analysis. Under the first model it could not be excluded, nor could it be excluded when the penetrance was reduced to 0.60. However, all analyses resulted in negative lod scores, arguing against a locus for schizophrenia in this region of chromosome 5.

Kaufmann et al. (1989) analyzed five DNA markers spanning the chromosome 5q11-q13 region in four North American pedigrees with 17 of 48 members diagnosed with schizophrenia or chronic schizoaffective disorder. The multipoint linkage analysis based on affected subjects only resulted in negative lod scores throughout the entire region examined and reaching −2.5 near the center of that region.

McGuffin et al. (1990) studied six multiplex pedigrees from Wales with a marker set containing the probes that appeared to be linked to schizophrenia in the Sherrington et al. (1988) study. The definitions of the affected phenotype included schizophrenia, schizophreniform disorder, delusional disorder, and depressive psychosis with mood-incongruent delusions. The genetic model assumed a dominant disease allele with a population frequency of 0.005, and 85% penetrance among heterozygotes and 100% among homozygotes (with 1% of homozygous normal individuals being affected). Negative lod scores were obtained across the entire region of interest, with most of the region formally excluded by lod scores lower than −2.0.

Aschauer et al. (1990) examined four loci, including two used by Sherrington et al. (1988), in seven North American pedigrees. When the pedigrees were analyzed with models of affection status similar to those used by Sherrington et al. (1988), no evidence of linkage was obtained over any of the region studied, and the majority of the region was excluded.

Iowa Multiplex Family Study

Thirty multiplex pedigrees of schizophrenia have been ascertained in Iowa through the Iowa Multiplex Family Study, and the analysis of six of these that are informative for linkage are reported here (see also Crowe et al. 1991).

The criterion for selecting pedigrees is a diagnosis of DSM-III-R (American Psychiatric Association 1987) schizophrenia in the proband and one relative, plus one additional relative with a schizophrenia spectrum diagnosis. The schizophrenia spectrum includes schizoaffective, schizophreniform, and schizotypal disorder. The pedigrees are extended through affected relatives and relatives who are obligate carriers by virtue of having affected relatives. Once the pedigree is extended, the entire nuclear family resulting from the extension is included in the study. Pedigrees with bilateral transmission or bipolar illness are excluded.

The principal interview instrument is the Comprehensive Assessment of Symptoms and History (CASH) (Andreasen 1985). In addition, the Schedule of Schizotypal Personalities (SSP) (Baron et al. 1981) and the Chapman scales (Chapman and Chapman 1980; Chapman et al. 1976, 1978) are given. The proband and first-degree relatives also receive a neurological examination, continuous performance task testing, smooth pursuit eye movement examination, and magnetic resonance imaging scan. The diagnoses for the linkage study are based on the CASH, SSP, and Chapman scales. They are made according to DSM-III-R criteria by consensus agreement of two psychiatrists blind to the DNA phenotype data.

Five DNA probes that map to the region of interest on chromosome 5 were used in the analyses: D5S21 (pJ0110H-C) detects two alleles with MspI; D5S76 (L599H-a) three alleles with TaqI; D5S6 (M4) three alleles with BamHI; D5S39 (p105-153a) two alleles with MspI and another two with XbaI, giving a four-allele haplotype; and D5S78 (p105-798Rb) two alleles with MspI. Probes were obtained from the American Type Culture Collection (Bethesda, Maryland). Methods employed for the DNA marker typing are described elsewhere (Crowe et al. 1991).

Linkage analyses were performed with the LINKAGE program, IBM PC version (Lathrop et al. 1985). Two-point analyses were performed with the MLINK program and three-point analyses with LINKMAP. The genetic model assumed autosomal dominant inheritance of a disease allele of frequency 0.008 and incomplete penetrance. Penetrances of 0.50,

0.70, and 0.90 were tested because they span the range of penetrances used in previous linkage studies of schizophrenia. In the multipoint analyses, D5S76 was arbitrarily set at 0 centiMorgans (cM), with D5S21 at −10 cM, D5S6 at +12 cM, and D5S39 at +15 cM (based on Keats et al. 1989). Because D5S78 was found not to contribute to the multipoint lod scores, it was not included in the multipoint analyses. A 1.5 ratio of female-to-male recombination was used in the multipoint analyses.

Three definitions of the affected phenotype were used. The first definition included only definite schizophrenia. The second definition included schizophrenia in addition to schizoaffective, schizophreniform, and schizotypal disorder. The third definition included all psychiatric diagnoses.

The six pedigrees comprised a total of 70 individuals and ranged in size from 7 to 17 persons. Genetic markers were typed on 55 individuals. Schizophrenia spectrum diagnoses were made on 19 individuals: schizophrenia, 11; schizotypal personality disorder, 5; schizoaffective disorder, 2; and schizophreniform disorder, 1. Nonspectrum diagnoses were made on 11 individuals and included unipolar depression, 7 (one psychotic); alcohol abuse disorder, 2; substance abuse disorder, 1; and obsessive-compulsive disorder, 1. An additional 3 relatives had schizophrenia spectrum diagnoses, which were considered in meeting inclusion criteria, but these persons were not included in the linkage analyses because marker data were not available on them.

Table 13–1 shows the two-point analyses assuming the schizophrenia

Table 13–1.   Lod scores for two-point analyses

Locus	Recombination fraction					
	.0001	.05	.10	.20	.30	.40
D5S21	−1.90	−1.41	−1.06	−0.57	−0.25	−0.07
D5S76	−7.63	−3.45	−2.27	−1.02	−0.39	−0.09
D5S6	−2.62	−1.61	−1.15	−0.57	−0.23	−0.05
D5S39	−1.63	−0.73	−0.39	−0.09	0.00	0.01
D5S78	−1.07	−0.68	−0.44	−0.19	−0.07	−0.01

Source. Reprinted from Crowe RR, Black DW, Wesner R, et al.: "Lack of Linkage to Chromosome 5q11-q13 Markers in Six Schizophrenia Pedigrees." *Archives of General Psychiatry* 48:357–361, 1991. Used with permission. Copyright 1991, American Medical Association.

spectrum to be the affected phenotype with a penetrance of 70%. All five markers generated negative lod scores, indicating that there is no evidence of linkage to any of the five. D5S76 excluded 20 cM of the region and the D5S6 locus was itself excluded; although the lod scores for the other three markers were negative, they did not exclude any of the region of interest.

Marker informativeness can be increased by combining markers in multipoint analyses. Accordingly, each pair of neighboring markers was included in a series of three-point analyses (a disease locus and two marker loci). Each successive set of three-point analyses was connected in Figure 13–1 to create a continuous lod score plot across the region of interest. Figure 13–1 shows that if the schizophrenia spectrum is assumed to be the disease phenotype with 70% penetrance, approximately 35 cM of the chromosome 5q11-q13 region can be excluded by a lod score of −2 or lower.

Additional analyses were conducted limiting the disease phenotype to schizophrenia as well as extending it to all Axis I diagnoses, assuming 50%, 70%, and 90% penetrance. As in the analyses already described,

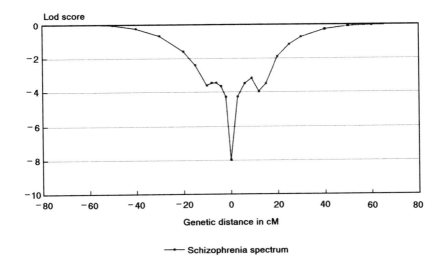

D5S21= −10; D5S6 = 0; D5S6 = 12; D5S39 = 15

Figure 13–1. Continuous lod score plot created by connecting a series of three-point analyses. Penetrance is 70%.

these analyses, too, resulted in negative lod scores across the entire region of interest.

It is important to address the question of whether any of the six pedigrees supported linkage to schizophrenia when considered individually. Table 13–2 presents the lod scores obtained at each of the four loci included in the multipoint analyses by individual family. The highest lod score obtained was 0.233 at the D5S39 locus in family 21. A lod score of this magnitude is most likely a chance result and, therefore, none of the pedigrees can be said to suggest linkage to a disease locus for schizophrenia.

Discussion

The dilemma posed by the discrepant results just reviewed has been a particularly vexing one because, coupled with the recent retraction of a high lod score for manic-depressive illness on chromosome 11 (Kelsoe et al. 1989), the success of linkage analysis as applied to psychiatry appears to hang in the balance. One is faced with reconciling a very high lod score supporting linkage to a schizophrenia locus on chromosome 5q11-q13 with a series of seven subsequent studies, not one of which has obtained positive lod scores for this region and many of which have excluded a schizophrenia locus from the region entirely. The question that must be addressed is whether any of the problems inherent in linkage analysis of complex traits can account for the inability to replicate a

Table 13–2. Lod scores for three-point analyses by pedigree at each locus

Pedigree	D5S21	D5S76	D5S6	D5S39
1	−0.797	−0.147	−0.235	−0.253
6	−0.837	−0.636	−0.772	−0.740
8	−0.151	−2.325	0.002	0.002
10	−1.115	−2.360	−1.357	−1.722
21	−0.151	0.093	0.209	0.233
22	−0.560	−2.580	−1.787	−1.012

Source. Reprinted from Crowe RR, Black DW, Wesner R, et al.: "Lack of Linkage to Chromosome 5q11-q13 Markers in Six Schizophrenia Pedigrees." *Archives of General Psychiatry* 48:357–361, 1991. Used with permission. Copyright 1991, American Medical Association.

true finding, and if not, whether they can account for lod scores as high as the ones reported in the absence of true linkage.

An obvious place to begin the analysis is with genetic heterogeneity, because that explanation was offered when early studies failed to replicate the original report of linkage (Lander 1988). Heterogeneity would seem to be a reasonable explanation because of the great likelihood that it would be present in a disease as diverse and complex as schizophrenia. The pedigrees that supported the linkage findings were drawn from Iceland in five cases and from England in two (Sherrington et al. 1988). Therefore, it is not surprising that the North Swedish kindred of Kennedy et al. (1988) might not replicate the finding, because it is a true population isolate and may be segregating a different gene for schizophrenia. However, Sherrington et al. (1988) pointed out that the genetic structure of Iceland is similar to that of northern England, northern Germany, and southern Sweden in allele frequencies. The genetic structure of Iceland, coupled with the fact that two pedigrees supporting linkage were from England, suggests that the finding should be replicable in European and North American Caucasian populations. Yet pedigrees from Scotland, Wales, and North America have failed to confirm linkage (Crowe et al. 1991; Detera-Wadleigh et al. 1990; Kaufmann et al. 1989; McGuffin et al. 1990; St. Clair et al. 1989).

It has been pointed out that genetic heterogeneity should be evident as heterogeneity *within* studies rather than as heterogeneity *across* studies (Risch 1990). Within studies, some pedigrees should support linkage while others should not. McGuffin et al. (1990) formally tested the published nonreplications and found no statistical evidence for genetic heterogeneity. Excluding the original report, there is no evidence for genetic heterogeneity either within or between studies. Finally, it should be remembered that genetic heterogeneity can be said to exist only when linkage to two different loci is confirmed; a nonreplication is simply a nonreplication (Risch 1990).

A second consideration in comparing the studies is diagnosis, because there was considerable variation across studies on this critical variable. The original report by Sherrington et al. (1988) found evidence of linkage to 1) schizophrenia, 2) schizophrenia plus five schizoid personality disorders (three of which have schizotypal features), and 3) all of the above plus another 10 relatives with other psychiatric diagnoses, including alcohol and drug abuse, depression, and phobic disorder. By contrast the Swedish pedigree contained only schizophrenia, and that with a high rate of catatonic features, rarely seen in schizophrenia today (Kennedy et al. 1988). Of the 15 pedigrees from Scotland, 7 contained bipolar illness (St. Clair et al. 1989). But even with this wide diagnostic variation it is difficult to account for the nonreplications. A number of the studies have used criteria similar to those of the original report, looking at varying levels of diagnostic certainty, without finding any support for linkage. Furthermore, when the pedigrees with bipolar illness were excluded from the Scottish sample, the analyses still failed to support linkage on chromosome 5 (St. Clair et al. 1989).

A third consideration in attempting to account for the differences is the genetic model employed in the analyses. This is an unlikely explanation because all of the studies assumed similar models—an autosomal dominant disease allele with a population frequency of approximately 0.8% and high penetrance. Several studies considered a range of genetic models, finding evidence for linkage with none. It seems particularly unlikely that the nonreplications are due to differences in model because the original report analyzed the data under a penetrance-free model and found support for linkage (Sherrington et al. 1988).

At this point, it appears that none of the factors considered here— genetic heterogeneity, choice of affected phenotype, and genetic model—can satisfactorily account for the discrepancy among studies. The next question to be considered is whether they can account for high lod scores in the absence of linkage.

The lod score is a parametric statistic based on the assumption that the pedigree can be correctly dichotomized into affected and unaffected phenotypes, and that the genetic model can be exactly specified. For classical Mendelian diseases such as Huntington's disease and cystic fibrosis, these criteria are fulfilled and the lod score accurately reflects the likelihood that the observed cosegregation of disease and marker could have occurred by chance alone. However, when these parameters cannot be accurately specified, the lod score loses its usual statistical meaning. In other words, one cannot conclude that a lod score of 3.0 is "high" because there is no way of knowing the likelihood of such a value occurring by chance. It is important to keep this principle in mind when interpreting what appear to be high lod scores for complex traits such as schizophrenia.

Uncertainty over the correct genetic model and correct definition of the affected phenotype can affect the lod score in another way, because it poses a research dilemma. Should the investigator perform a single analysis and risk missing real linkage because of erroneous assumptions, or should he or she perform a set of analyses and risk inflating the lod score by making multiple comparisons? Sherrington et al. (1988) chose the second alternative and considered three definitions of affected phenotype, testing six penetrances, ranging from 50% to 100%, on each phenotype. Thus, 18 analyses were performed. As a way out of this dilemma, Ott (1990) proposed carrying out simulations on the pedigree set to arrive at a revised critical lod score value that allows for multiple comparisons. For example, when such simulations are performed on the seven pedigrees of Sherrington et al. (1988), a lod score criterion of 3.625 for concluding linkage is suggested.

Another means of escape from the uncertainty over the statistical analysis of the data is the use of an analysis that is free of assumptions about phenotype and genetic model. The linkage analysis can be restricted to cases that everyone would agree should fit the affected phenotype, thus ignoring pedigree members who are either unaffected or affected with some other illness. But the freedom comes at a price. That price is a considerable loss of statistical power to detect linkage. Sherrington et al. (1988) reanalyzed their data under a "zero penetrance" model, which ignores unaffected pedigree members in computing the lod score, and a lod score of 2.45 was obtained. Although this is still supportive of linkage, it is well below even the conventional critical value of 3.0.

Finally, it should be remembered that the lod scores obtained for schizophrenia and the schizophrenia spectrum in the Sherrington et al. (1988) study were 3.22 and 4.33, respectively. The highest lod score (6.49) resulted from the inclusion of disorders that family, twin, and adoption studies have not placed in the schizophrenia spectrum. If consideration is limited to the analyses based on a definition of the schizophrenia spectrum that would be broadly agreed upon (Weeks et al. 1990), the lod scores are not impressively high in view of the foregoing considerations. Once a linkage has been firmly established, it would be appropriate to define the spectrum on the basis of which diagnoses carry the linked marker allele. But it is circular reasoning to conclude that a group of disorders are genetically related to the core disease because they maximize the lod score.

Conclusion

What lessons have we learned from linkage research in schizophrenia and other psychiatric diseases? Perhaps the most important lesson is that the lod score, no matter how high, does not waive the requirement for replication of the result. Confirmation of linkage still requires a critical lod score by two independent laboratories. Recent experience has demonstrated how important this principle is in psychiatric research because of the complex nature of the disorders being studied.

However, since other investigators may not have access to the population in which the linkage was reported, it is important that the investigators reporting the linkage replicate the finding in their own material. This can be done in several ways. One strategy is to extend the pedigrees to include additional branches. If the original finding represents true linkage the lod score should increase; otherwise it should decrease. The power of this strategy was recently illustrated by the findings of Kelsoe et al. (1989). A second strategy is to study additional pedigrees from the same population. If the original lod score represents true linkage, it should be replicable in this way. A third strategy is to examine additional genetic markers in the region of interest. Turning previously uninformative branches of the pedigrees into informative ones with new markers has the same effect as extending the pedigrees.

Another lesson learned from linkage research is that definitions of the affected phenotype and the genetic models should be specified in advance. Reported lod scores should be based on these prior hypotheses and not exploratory analyses. The latter may lead to new hypotheses to be tested in future studies, but should be clearly labeled as exploratory. Just as linkage findings should be based on prior hypotheses, attempts to replicate the finding must be based on the same considerations. If studies failing to replicate a linkage finding report only the analyses that minimize the lod score and exclude the greatest amount of genome, the problems of resolving these investigations will only be compounded.

Molecular genetics provides a powerful new strategy for studying disease. It is especially appealing to psychiatry because of the difficulty of studying the brain in affected individuals by traditional methods. However, molecular genetics can be only as powerful as the clinical assessments and genetic assumptions that go into it. Therefore, it should not be surprising that problems have arisen in applying the method to psychiatric disease. Fortunately, the power of the method includes the ability to validate or repudiate provisional findings. There is every reason to believe that we will emerge from this period of difficulties with more rigorous methodologies for applying molecular genetics to psychiatric disease that will allow the fulfillment of its ultimate promise of delivering the genetic code causing mental illness.

References

American Psychiatric Association: Diagnostic and Statistical Manual of Mental Disorders, 3rd Edition, Revised. Washington, DC, American Psychiatric Association, 1987

Anderson MP, Gregory RJ, Thompson S, et al: Demonstration that CFTR is a chloride channel by alteration of its anion selectivity. Science 253:202–205, 1991

Andreasen NC: Comprehensive Assessment of Symptoms and History (CASH). Iowa City, The University of Iowa, 1985

Aschauer HN, Aschauer-Treiber G, Isenberg KE, et al: No evidence for linkage between chromosome 5 markers and schizophrenia. Hum Hered 40:109–115, 1990

Baron M, Asnis L, Gruen R: The schedule for schizotypal personalities (SSP): a diagnostic interview for schizotypal features. Psychiatry Res 4:213–228, 1981

Bassett AS, Jones BD, McGillivray BC, et al: Partial trisomy chromosome 5 cosegregating with schizophrenia. Lancet 1:799–800, 1988

Chapman LJ, Chapman JP: Scales for rating psychotic and psychotic-like experiences as continua. Schizophr Bull 6:476–489, 1980

Chapman LJ, Chapman JP, Rowland ML: Scales for physical and social anhedonia. J Abnorm Psychol 85:374–382, 1976

Chapman LJ, Chapman JP, Rowland ML: Body-image aberration in schizophrenia. J Abnorm Psychol 87:399–407, 1978

Crowe RR, Black DW, Wesner R, et al: Lack of linkage to chromosome 5q11-q13 markers in six schizophrenia pedigrees. Arch Gen Psychiatry 48:357–361, 1991

Detera-Wadleigh SD, Goldin LR, Sherrington R, et al: Exclusion of linkage to 5q11-q13 in families with schizophrenia and other psychiatric disorders. Nature 340:391–393, 1990

Kaufmann CA, DeLisi LE, Lehner T, et al: Physical mapping, linkage analysis of a susceptibility locus for schizophrenia on chromosome 5q. Schizophr Bull 15:441–452, 1989

Keats B, Ott J, Conneally M: Report of the committee on linkage and gene order, in Human Gene Mapping 10: New Haven Conference (1989): Tenth International Workshop on Human Gene Mapping. Edited by Kidd KK, Klinger HP, Ruddle FH. New York, Karger, 1989, pp 459–502

Kelsoe JR, Ginns EI, Egeland JA, et al: Re-evaluation of the linkage relationship between chromosome 11p loci and the gene for bipolar affective disorder in the Old Order Amish. Nature 342:238–243, 1989

Kennedy JL, Guiffra LA, Moises HW, et al: Evidence against linkage of schizophrenia to markers on chromosome 5 in a northern Swedish pedigree. Nature 336:167–170, 1988

Kerem B, Rommens JM, Buchanan JA, et al: Identification of the cystic fibrosis gene: genetic analysis. Science 245:1073–1080, 1989

Lander ES: Splitting schizophrenia. Nature 336:105–106, 1988

Lathrop GM, Lalouel JM, Julier C, et al: Multilocus linkage analysis in humans: detection of linkage and estimation of recombination. Am J Hum Genet 37:482–498, 1985

Martin JB: Molecular genetics: applications to the clinical neurosciences. Science 238:765–772, 1987

McGillivray BC, Bassett AS, Langlois S, et al: Familial 5q11.2-11.3 segmental duplication cosegregating with multiple anomalies, including schizophrenia. Am J Med Genet 35:10–13, 1990

McGuffin P, Sargeant M, Gillian H, et al: Exclusion of a schizophrenia susceptibility gene from the chromosome 5q11-q13 region: new data and a reanalysis of previous reports. Am J Hum Genet 47:524–535, 1990

Ott J: Genetic linkage and complex diseases: a comment. Genet Epidemiol 7:35–36, 1990

Pardes H, Kaufmann CA, Pincus JA, et al: Genetics and psychiatry: past discoveries, current dilemmas, and future directions. Am J Psychiatry 146:435–443, 1989

Riordan JR, Rommens JM, Kerem B, et al: Identification of the cystic fibrosis gene: cloning and characterization of complementary DNA. Science 245:1066–1072, 1989

Risch N: Genetic linkage and complex diseases, with special reference to psychiatric disorders. Genet Epidemiol 7:3–16, 1990

Rommens JM, Iannuzzi MC, Kerem B, et al: Identification of the cystic fibrosis gene: chromosome walking and jumping. Science 245:1059–1065, 1989

Sherrington R, Brynjolfsson J, Petursson H, et al: Localization of a susceptibility locus for schizophrenia on chromosome 5. Nature 336:164–167, 1988

St. Clair D, Blackwood D, Muir W, et al: No linkage of chromosome 5q11-q13 markers to schizophrenia in Scottish families. Nature 339:305–309, 1989

Suarez BK, Cox NJ: Linkage analysis for psychiatric disorders, I: basic concepts. Psychiatric Developments 3:219–243, 1985

Tsui L-C, Buchwald M, Barker D, et al: Cystic fibrosis locus defined by a genetically linked polymorphic DNA marker. Science 230:1054–1057, 1985

Wainwright BJ, Scambler PJ, Schmidtke J, et al: Localization of cystic fibrosis locus to human chromosome 7cen-q22. Nature 318:384–385, 1985

Weeks DE, Brzustowicz L, Squires-Wheeler E, et al: Report of a workshop on genetic linkage studies in schizophrenia. Schizophr Bull 16:673–686, 1990

White R, Caskey CT: The human as an experimental system in molecular genetics. Science 240:1483–1488, 1988

White RS, Woodward M, Leppert M, et al: A closely linked genetic marker for cystic fibrosis. Nature 318:382–384, 1985

Index

Abnormal Involuntary Movement
  Scale, 80
Absence of services, 203
Abstract thinking, diminished
  capacity for, 9
Activity, intrinsic, of partial dopamine
  receptor agonists, 164
Acute phase, psychosocial treatment
  strategies for, 206
Adoption studies, 190
Adoptive plateau phase, psychosocial
  treatment strategies for, 206
ADP
  energy metabolism and, 228
  in vivo studies of, 229
  ^{31}P NMR of, **224,** 224
Advocacy, 30
Affect
  disorders of, 222. *See also* Affective
    blunting
  flattening of. *See* Affective blunting
  inappropriate, 57
Affective blunting
  assessment of, **58,** 58–59
  disturbed function in, **56**
  factor analysis studies of, **57**
  heterogeneity of, 52
  modeling of, 54
  as negative symptom, 57
  in schizophrenic patient, 9, 16

Affective style, in family, 192–193
Aftercare programs, 17
Aging
  Alzheimer's disease and, 236
  of brain, ^{31}P NMR animal studies
    of, 226–228
  normal, schizophrenia and, 236
  normal brain development and,
    232–233
  schizophrenia and, 236
Agrammatism, 54
Agranulocytosis, clozapine and, 8, 10,
  17
(+)-AJ76, 166, **167**
Alogia
  disturbed function in, **56**
  factor analysis studies of, **57**
  as negative symptom, 57
Alzheimer's disease
  long-term neuroleptic therapy, D_2
    receptors and, 125
  membrane abnormalities in, 222
  normal aging and, 236
  similarities with schizophrenia, 9,
    14
Ambivalence, 8
Amphetamine, 176–177
Amygdala
  cholecystokinin in, 131
  dopamine in, 131

Page numbers printed in **boldface** *type refer to tables or figures.*

Amygdala *(continued)*
  homovanillic acid in, 131
  lesions of, 95
Angel dust (phencyclidine; PCP),
  169–170
Anhedonia
  disturbed function in, **56**
  factor analysis studies of, **57**
  heterogeneity of, 52
  as negative symptom, 57
  in schizophrenic patient, 11–12
Animal models
  of antipsychotic therapeutic
    efficacy, 54
  brain development/aging studies
    of, 226–228
  D1 receptor studies in, 127
  lack of, 53
  primate, 54
  strongest, 54
Anterior cingulate gyrus, serotonin
  receptors and, 181
Antidepressants, long-term treatment
  with, 163
Antiparkinsonian drugs, long-term
  treatment with, 163
Antipsychotics
  long-term treatment with, 163
  PET studies of dopamine receptors
    and, 151–153, **152**
  postsynaptic dopamine blockade
    and, 166
AP-5, 168
Asylum services, treatment effect
  and, **198**
ATP
  in autistic patients, 235
  brain levels of, 228
  decreased utilization of, 235
  energy metabolism and, 228
  in vivo studies of, 229
  ^{31}P NMR study of, **224,** 224
Attention, 50

Attention deficits
  disturbed function in, **56**
  factor analysis studies of, **57**
  in genetic studies of children, 96
  as negative symptom, 57
  subcortical and cortical
    dysfunction and, 96
Auditory processing, 50
Autistic patients
  in vivo ^{31}P NMR studies of, 235
  PET studies of, 235
Autonomy, 41
Autoreceptor antagonists,
  preferential, 166
Autoreceptors, dopaminergic, 164,
  166
Autosomal dominant disease, 256
Avolition
  disturbed function in, **56**
  factor analysis studies of, **57**
  heterogeneity of, 52
  as negative symptom, 57

Basal ganglia
  classic neuropathological studies,
    130
  constituents of, 124. *See also specific
    basal ganglia regions*
  neurotransmitters in, 127, **129**
  non-D2 receptors in, **128**
  number of D2 receptors in, **125**
  postmortem studies of, 124–131
Behavior
  bizarre
    developmental aspects of, 40–41
    disturbed function in, **56**
    factor analysis studies of, **57**
  brain regulation and, 93–94
  disorganized, 57
  goal-directed, disorganization of, 94
Behavioral imaging, 99–100
Biological psychiatry
  diagnostic fit and, 34–35

prognosis and, 35–36
vs. psychodynamic approach, 32–34
Biplot algorithm, of diagnostic
    categories, 34–35
Bipolar disorder, 249–250
Birth weight, co-twin control method
    and, 109–110, **110**
Bizarre behavior. *See* Behavior, bizarre
Bleuler, E., 37
Brain. *See also specific brain structures*
    aging, ^{31}P NMR animal studies of,
        226–228
    anterior lesions of, 94
    ATP levels, in autistic patients, 235
    development
        ^{31}P NMR animal studies of,
            226–228
        periods of, 225–226
    disease, schizophrenia as, 28
    imaging studies of, **112**
    normal development, aging, and,
        232–233
    regional dysfunction of, 98–99
    regional energy metabolism in,
        148–150
    regional function, behavior and,
        93–94
    regional hypotheses in
        neuropsychology, 96
    structure
        co-twin study of, **110–111, 112,
            113**
        lesions of, 94
Brain stem
    neuropathology studies, 136
    postmortem studies of, 135–136
Broca's aphasia, vs. schizophrenia, 54
76-Bromospiperone, 150–151
Brooks, George, 212–213

California Verbal Learning Test, 95
Cardiac malformations, 114

CASH (Comprehensive Assessment
    of Symptoms and History), 55,
    80, 251
Catecholamine metabolites, in
    nucleus accumbens of
    schizophrenic patients, **129**
Catecholamines
    in nucleus accumbens of
        schizophrenic patients, **129**
    source of, 135
Caudate
    D1 receptor studies, 127
    D2 receptors in, 124
    number of D2 receptors, **125**
CCK. *See* Cholecystokinin (CCK)
Cerebral blood flow
    in frontal cortex, negative
        symptoms and, **84, 85–86**
    measurement of, 69
    regional, 137
    SPECT studies of, 69, **70–75**
    ^{133}Xe method for, 80
Cerebral blood metabolism,
    measurement of, 69
Cerebral cortex
    corticostriatal pathway of, 168–169,
        169, 170
    postmortem studies of, 133–135,
        134
Cerebral ventricular size, co-twin
    control method and, **110–111,
    112, 113**
Cerebrospinal fluid norepinephrine,
    181–182
Change periods, psychosocial
    treatment strategies for, 206
Chemotherapy, 210–211
Childhood, premorbid, 6
Chlorpromazine, 174
Cholecystokinin (CCK)
    in amygdala, 131
    in cerebral cortex, 133, **134**
    in hippocampus, 131–132

Cholecystokinin (CCK) *(continued)*
  in thalamus, 136
Chromosome 5q11-q13, 248, 249, 250
Clinical description, **55**, 55
Clinical goals, 199
Clinical outcome dimensions, 199
Clinicians, advice for, 16–17
Clonidine, 170
Clopenthixol, 180
Clozapine
  agranulocytosis and, 17
  atypical neuroleptic development
    and, 178–179
  D_1 and D_2 receptors and, 183
  D_4 receptor and, 177
  depolarization blockade model
    and, 179
  efficacy of, 175
  in fenfluramine challenge test,
    180–181
  potency of, 182
  preclinical studies, 179
  prolactin and, 179
  removal of, 10
  serotonergic systems and, 180
  side effects of, 8
Co-twin control method, birth weight
    and, 109–110, **110**
Co-twin dead twins, 114–115
Cognition
  impairment of, 9, 10
  normal processes of, 50
Communicative deviance, 192–193
Community-based treatment, 23, 24
Comprehensive Assessment of
    Symptoms and History (CASH),
    55, 80, 251
Computed tomography (CT)
  of brain, 10
  of third ventricle enlargement,
    133
  of ventricular size, 110–111, **112,**
    113

Computers, for training and
    relearning, 17
Concordance rates, for
    schizophrenia, **106, 107,** 107
Configurations, psychological and
    neurophysiological, 37–38
Congenital anomalies, 6, 114
Continuous Performance Test, 79
Continuous reevaluation strategy, in
    psychosocial treatment, 205
Control mechanisms, 40
Cortical cerebral metabolic rate, 149
Corticostriatal pathway, 168–169, **169,**
    170
Costs of schizophrenia, 26–28
Course of disorder, 38–40
Criminal justice system,
    deinstitutionalization and, 26–27
Critical feelings, 13–14
CT. *See* Computed tomography (CT)
Cultural factors, 190–191
Cystic fibrosis, 246, 256
Cytidine diphosphocholine, 225
Cytidine diphosphoethanolamine, 225

D_1 receptors
  antipsychotic drug therapy and, 153
  clozapine and, 153–154
  studies of, 127
  typical vs. atypical neuroleptics
    and, 182–183
D_2 receptors
  in basal ganglia, 124, 128–129
  in caudate, 124
  clozapine treatment and, **152,**
    152–153
  density
    bimodal distribution of, 126–127
    in neuroleptic-treated
        Huntington's disease, 126
    in neuroleptic-treated senile
        dementia, 126
    positive symptoms and, 126

in nucleus accumbens, 136
number of
in basal ganglia, **125**
in limbic system, **125**
PET of, 150–153, **152**
in putamen, 124
in striatum, 136
in striatum of drug-naive
schizophrenic patients,
237–238
in substantia nigra, 135
D4 receptors
and clozapine, 177
Data interpretation, methodological
issues in, 96–98
Decade of the Brain, 31, 42, 51
Deinstitutionalization
criminal justice system and,
26–27
Dix, Dorothea and, 213
homelessness and, 24
ongoing implementation of, 23
Delusions
in affected phenotype, 250
content of, 15–16, 42
disturbed function in, **56**
evaluation of, 48
factor analysis studies of, **57**
as positive symptom, 57
in schizophrenic patient, 8, 9–10
Dementia praecox
description of, 50
loss of will and, 37
normal aging and, 236
subtypes, 35
Demoralization, 33
Depression, 7
Depressive psychosis, with mood-
incongruent delusions, 250
Descriptive psychiatry
importance of, 41–42
vs. neuroscience, 32–34, 42
Development, 40–41

Diabetes mellitus, 121
Diagnosis, variations, linkage analysis
studies and, 255–256
"Diagnosis is prognosis," 35
Diagnostic categories, 34–35
Diagnostic concepts, 36–38
Diagnostic criteria, 108–109
Dihydroxyphenylacetic acid
(DOPAC), **129**
Disabilities, mental, 21–22
Disappointment, 11
Disorganized speech, 48, 50, 52, 57
Dix, Dorothea, 209, 212–213
DNA, double helix structure of,
219
L-Dopa, 176–177
DOPAC (dihydroxyphenylacetic
acid), **129**
Dopamine
in amygdala, 131
in nucleus accumbens, **129**, 130
projections, language dysfunction
and, 54
receptors. See D1 receptors; D2
receptors; D4 receptors
Dopamine agonists
shortcomings of, 162–163
time course of response and,
176–177
Dopamine hypothesis, 150, 160,
177–178
Dopamine-to-norepinephrine ratios,
in thalamus, 136
Dopaminergic antagonists, 163
Dopaminergic supersensitivity,
clozapine and, 179
Dopaminergic system, nervous
pathway interactions,
pharmacologic manipulation of,
167–170, **168, 169**
Dose-response relationships, 174
Drugs. See Medications; specific drugs
DSM-III, multiaxial diagnosis, 36

Educational attainment, data
    interpretation and, 97
Efficacy, of neuroleptics, 173–175
Electroconvulsive therapy, 8
Emotional connectedness, loss of,
    9–10
Emotional emptiness, 54
Emotions, expressed, in family, 192,
    193–194
End states, psychosocial treatment
    strategies for, 207
Endorphins, in hypothalamus, 131
Entorhinal cortex, 132
    cytoarchitectonic abnormalities in,
        133
Environment
    etiology and, 14, 53
    risk of schizophrenia, twins and,
        109–115, **110, 112, 113, 114,**
        115
Enzymes, high PME levels in brain
    development and, 226–227
Etiology
    diversity of, 52–53
    environmental factors and, 14, 53
    factors in, 14–15
    genetic factors, 53
    patient history and, 6
    psychological factors, 14–15
    social factors, 14–15
Evaluation strategy, in psychosocial
    treatment, 204–205
Executive functions
    deficits, 94
    psychometric tests of, 94–95
Expressed emotion, in family, 13,
    192, 193–194
Extrapyramidal side effects
    antidopaminergic activity and,
        180
    dopamine receptor blockade and,
        164–165
    heterogeneity of, 177

Facial dysmorphism, 248
Factor analysis studies
    of negative symptoms, **57,** 57
    of positive symptoms, **57,** 57
Family(ies). *See also* Parents
    costs of schizophrenia on, 27
    hospitalizations and, 191
    observations of, 16
    in schizophrenic psychopathology,
        192–194
    support of, 11, 13
    in treatment program, 16–17
    violence in, 27
Family/consumer movement, 25
Family therapy, 207–209, **208**
Father, of schizophrenic son,
    experience of, 6–12
Federal entitlement programs, 24,
    25, 28–29
Fenfluramine challenge test, 180–181
Fiscal responsibility for care, 28–29
Freud, Sigmund, 37
Frontal lobe
    hypothesis. *See* Hypofrontality
        hypothesis
    interconnectivity with diencephalic
        limbic and reticular
        structures, 96
    metabolism, SPECT studies of,
        70–75
    neural substrates of, 62–69
    postmortem studies of, 135
Frustration, subjective, 54
Functional analysis of deficits, 98–99
Functional neuroimaging, 69

Gamma-aminobutyric acid (GABA)
    in cerebral cortex, **134**
    in thalamus, 135–136
GENCAP program, 229
Genetic epistemology, 33
Genetic heterogeneity, linkage
    analysis and, 255

Genetic model, 254–257
Genetics of schizophrenia, 53
Gliosis, 133, 136
Global Assessment Scale, 80
Globus pallidus, 124, 127
Globus pallidus interna, 130
Glucose metabolism
  in neocortical and central brain
    regions, 148–149
  regional brain, during neuroleptic
    treatment, 150
Glutamate, 133–134
Glutamatergic/aspartergic
  corticostriatal pathway, 168–169,
  169, 170
Glutamic acid dehydrogenase, 135,
  136
Glycerol 3-phosphocholine (GPC),
  224, 224, 226
Glycerol 3-phosphoethanolamine
  (GPE), **224,** 224, 226
Goal, 198–199
Goal-directed behavior, 37–38
α-GP, 226
GPC (glycerol 3-phosphocholine),
  224, 224, 226
GPE (glycerol 3-phospho-
  ethanolamine), **224,** 224, 226
Grief, 5, 8, 9

Hallucinations
  auditory, inability to model, 53
  disturbed function in, **56**
  evaluation of, 48
  factor analysis studies of, **57**
  heterogeneity of, 52
  lessening of, 38
  as positive symptom, 57
Haloperidol
  blood levels vs. clinical response,
    174–175
  D_2-to-S_2 ratio, 180

neuroleptic threshold hypothesis
  and, 174
Halstead Category Test, 96
Halstead-Reitan neuropsychological
  battery, 94
Hamilton Rating Scale for
  Depression, 80
Handedness, in twins, 113–114
Hearing voices, 41–42, 50
Heterogeneity
  clinical, 52
    standard deviation and, 52–53
  of drug response, 173–174
  genetic, linkage analysis and, 255
Hexose 6-phosphate (H6P), **224,** 224
High-energy phosphate metabolism
  in aging, 232–233
  in normal brain development,
    232–233
Hippocampus
  cholecystokinin in, 131–132
  lesions of, 95
  neurochemical studies of, 131, 132
  twin studies of, 111
Homelessness, 24, 28
Homovanillic acid (HVA)
  in amygdala, 131
  in nucleus accumbens of
    schizophrenic patients, **129**
  time-dependent changes in, 178
Hospitalization, need for, 36
Humanistic goals, 199
Humanitarian outcome dimensions,
  201–202
Humiliation, 10, 11
Huntington's disease
  lod scores for, 256
  long-term neuroleptic therapy, D_2
    receptors and, 125
  membrane abnormalities in, 222
  neuroleptic-treated, D_2 receptor
    density in, 126
HVA. *See* Homovanillic acid (HVA)

6-Hydroxydopamine theory, 136
5-Hydroxyindoleacetic acid, 127
α-Hydroxylase, 181
Hypervigilance,
    amphetamine-induced, 53–54
Hypofrontality hypothesis, 100–101
    drug-naive schizophrenic patients
        and, 79–81, **82–83**, 84
    evidence of, 222–223
    negative symptoms and, 79, 84
    from PET studies, 69, **76–78**
    from SPECT studies, 69, **70–75**
    imaging modalities for, 69
    selective impairment of, 98
Hypothalamus, 131, 136

Imaging modalities. *See also specific
    imaging modalities,* 69
In vivo neuroimaging
    of hypothalamic abnormalities, 133
    of limbic system abnormalities, 132
    with postmortem studies, 122, 123
Incidence of schizophrenia, 26
Indoleamine, 135
Inorganic orthophosphate (Pi), 226,
    227
    decreased production of, 235
    energy metabolism and, 228
    in vivo studies of, 229
    ^{31}P NMR study of, **224,** 224
    ratio to phosphocreatine, 229
Inositol 1,4,5-triphosphate, 225
Instrumental functioning outcome
    dimensions, 200
Insurance, private, for mental
    disorders, 23
Integration, of psychosocial and drug
    treatment, 205
Intellectual emptiness, brain
    abnormalities and, 50
Internal suffering, 3
Interpersonal psychotherapy, 211

Intrinsic activity, of partial dopamine
    receptor agonists, 164
Intrinsic efficacy, of partial dopamine
    receptor agonists, 163, 164
Iowa Multiplex family study, **251–254,
    252, 253**
Isolation, tendency toward, 7

Kainic acid, 133
Knowledge base, 54–55
Kraepelin, E., 35, 37, 49–50

Language
    abnormal perception/production,
        brain structure/function, and,
        50
    circuitry for, 54
    concreteness of, 9
    expressive, loss of, 9
    richness, loss of, 9
Language tests, 96
Late prodromal phase, psychosocial
    treatment strategies for, 206
Laterality
    handedness and, 113–114
    hypothesis of, 100
    related disorders of, twins and, 113
Learning tests, temporal lobe
    hypothesis and, 98
Length of illness, prior to drug
    therapy, treatment outcome and,
    176
Leukotomized patients
    lesion, magnetic resonance scan of,
        64
    neuropsychological functioning in,
        66–69, 67, 68, 69
    positive vs. negative symptoms in,
        63–64, **65, 66**
    study of, 62–69
Life events, stressful, 191–192
Ligands, for PET scan studies,
    150–151

Limbic system
  components of, 131
  number of D₂ receptors, **125**
  postmortem studies of, 131–133
Linkage analysis, 257–258
  computer programs for, 251–252
  genetic heterogeneity and, 255
  lod scores
    for three-point analysis, **253,**
      253, **254**
    for two-point analysis, **252,**
      252–253
  multipoint, 249
  for phenotypic classification,
    248–249
  principles of, 245–248
  with zero penetrance model, 256
LINKAGE program, 251
LINKMAP program, 251
Literature review, of molecular
  genetic research, 248–250
Lithium, 8
Lod scores, 246
  for three-point analysis, **253,** 253,
    254
  for two-point analysis, **252,** 252–253
Long-term impact of schizophrenia,
  28
Longitudinal processes, 38
Lorentzian peaks, 229, **231**
Loss
  of emotional connectedness, 9–10
  of expectations, 9
  of feelings/emotions, 16
  sense of, 5, 8, 9, 11
  types, for families of schizophrenic
    patient, 27–28
Loxapine, 8
Luria-Nebraska neuropsychological
  battery, 94

Magnetic resonance imaging (MRI)
  of cerebral ventricular size, 111

limbic system abnormalities, 132
³¹P nuclear magnetic resonance.
  See Phosphorus–31 nuclear
    magnetic resonance
  of temporal lobe gray matter, 135
Mainstreaming, 25
Mammillary bodies, 131
MAO (monoamine oxidase), 110
Maudsley Twin Register, 107–110, **108**
Measurements
  importance of, 37
  repeated, 38
Medial temporal lobe
  lesions of, 95
  volume of, 133
Medicaid
  eligibility, 25
  fiscal responsibility and, 29
  importance of, 22
  optional services, 24
  reimbursable services, 24
Medications. *See also specific medications*
  effects on evaluation of
    phenomenology, 52
  family observations about, 16
  for fostering socialization, 210–211
  new, development of, 17
  withdrawal of, 10
Medulla, 135
Membrane phospholipid metabolism
  in aging, 232–233
  in normal brain development,
    232–233
  in schizophrenia, evidence for,
    222–223
  in schizophrenic vs. control
    subjects, 233–235
Memory, 50
Memory tests, temporal lobe
  hypothesis and, 98
Mental health system, 22
Mental illness
  biological causes of, 31–32

Mental illness *(continued)*
  categories of, 14
  cost of, 26–28
  disability of, 21
  homelessness and, 24
  in prisons, 27
  stigma of, 10
  studying, sequential program for,
    55, 55–56
Mental institutions, long-term care
  in, 25
Mesencephalon, 135
3-Methoxy-4-hydroxyphenylglycol
  (MHPG), **129,** 130
N-Methyl-D-aspartate (NMDA), 132,
  134
Methylphenidate, 176–177
[11]C-*N*-Methylspiperone, 150–151
MHPG (3-methoxy-4-
  hydroxyphenylglycol), **129,** 130
Midfrontal gyrus, serotonin receptors
  and, 181
Mixed agonist/antagonist, 164. *See
  also* Partial dopamine receptor
  agonists
MK-212, 180
MK-801, 168, 169–170
MLINK program, 251
Model development. *See also* Animal
  models
  neural aspects of, problems in, **53,**
    53–55
  phenomenologic aspects of, **51,**
    51–53
Molecular genetic research, 219–220
  linkage analysis, 245–248
  literature review, 248–250
  [31]P nuclear magnetic resonance
    studies of. *See* Phosphorus–31
    nuclear magnetic resonance
Molecular genetics. *See also* Linkage
  analysis
Monoamine oxidase (MAO), 110

Monoaminergic transmitter amines,
  150
Moratorium phase, psychosocial
  treatment strategies for, 206
Mortality, preoccupation with, 8
Mothers, schizophrenogenic, 14
Mourning
  for dead child, 5
  without end, 5, 8, 9, 10
MRI. *See* Magnetic resonance imaging
  (MRI)
Multipoint linkage analysis, 249
Myotonia dystrophy, 222

National Alliance for the Mentally Ill
  (NAMI), 4, 10
Natural history
  prognostic factors and, **196,**
    196–198, **198**
  treatment effect and, **197**
Nature vs. nurture controversy, 105
Negative symptoms, 36
  central noradrenergic pathway
    deterioration and, 181
  cerebral blood flow in frontal
    cortex and, 84, **85–86**
  factor analysis studies of, **57,** 57
  hypofrontality and, 79, 84
  in leukotomized patients, 63–64,
    65, 66
  listing of, **56,** 57
  neuroleptics and, 10
  prefrontal cortex and, 59, **61,** 61–62
  SAPS, reliability coefficients for
    items in, **60**
  in schizophrenic patient, 8, 9
  standardized evaluation techniques
    for, 57–58
Neural mechanisms
  identification of, 49–50
  in model development, problems
    of, **53,** 53–55
Neural substrates, 54

Neurobiology
  emerging technologies, 122
  traditional methods, 121–122
Neurochemistry
  of hypothalamus, 131
  postmortem changes in, 123. *See also* Postmortem studies
Neurohumoral transmission, discovery of, 161
Neuroimaging studies, 95. *See also specific neuroimaging techniques*
Neuroleptic threshold hypothesis, 174
Neuroleptics, 8
  antidepressant actions of, 166
  atypical, 178
  blood levels vs. clinical response, 174–175
  development of, 159
  dopamine hypothesis and, 177–178
  effects on cerebral cortex, 135
  efficacy of, 173–175
  equal efficacy of, 175
  high expressed emotion families and, 193
  long-term therapy, D2 receptors and, 125
  maintenance, life event stress, and, 192
  negative symptoms and, 10
  nonresponders, 12–13
  therapeutic window of, 175
  time course of response, 176–177
  treatment, regional brain glucose metabolism in, 150
  typical vs. atypical, 160, 178–183
Neuromodulators, 127
Neuropathology. *See also* Etiology
  postmortem changes in, 123
Neuropharmacology, 161–170
Neurophysiological description, **55**
Neurophysiology
  configurations, 37–38
  techniques of, 56

Neuropsychological batteries
  application to schizophrenia, 95–96
  fixed, 94
  flexible, 94
  measured dimensions of, 94–95
  nature of, 94–95
Neuropsychological description, **55**
Neuropsychology
  techniques of, 56
  testing, 100. *See also* Neuropsychological batteries
Neuroscience, vs. descriptive psychiatry, 32–34, 42
Neurotensin, 133
Neurotransmitters
  in basal ganglia of schizophrenic patients, 127, **129**
  in synapse, 161
Neurotrophic agents, potential therapeutic effects of, 238
Nicolet data station, 229
Nicotinamide adenine dinucleotide phosphate (NADP), **224**, 224
NIMH, The National Plan for Schizophrenia Research, 29–30
NMDA (*N*-methyl-D-aspartate), 132, **134**
NMDA-receptor agonist, 170
NMDA receptors, 168
Noncompliance, 40
Non-D2 receptors, in basal ganglia of schizophrenic patients, **128**
Nonresponders, 12–13
Norepinephrine
  in nucleus accumbens, **129,** 130
  pathophysiology of schizophrenia and, 181–182
  in pons, 135
Normalization, 25
Nucleotide triphosphates, **224**, 224
Nucleus accumbens, 124
  D2 receptors, 136

Nucleus accumbens *(continued)*
  dopamine concentration in
    schizophrenia, 127–128
  number of D2 receptors, **125**
Null hypothesis, 246

Obstetric complications, twins and,
    114
Occupational functioning, 36
On-off phenomenon, 163
Onset of illness, 7
Outcome
  predictors of, **191**
  studies, two-point analyses of, 38
Overinvolvement, of parents, 13–14

Parahippocampal gyrus, 132
Parahippocampal gyrus, pre–α-cells
    in, 237
Parental communications, 192
Parental neglect, 14
Parents. *See also* Family(ies)
  father, experience of, 6–12
  intense feelings of, 5
  mothers, schizophrenogenic, 14
  overinvolvement of, 13–14
Parkinson's disease
  chronic treatment of, 163
  vs. schizophrenia, 54
Partial dopamine receptor agonists,
    163–165, **165**
Pathogenesis, 17
Pathophysiology of schizophrenia,
    norepinephrine and, 181–182
PCP (phencyclidine; angel dust),
    169–170
PCr. *See* Phosphocreatine (PCr)
PDE. *See* Phosphodiester (PDE)
Pedigrees, multiplex, **251–254, 252,
    253, 254**
Penetrance, 247–248, 251–252
Perception, abnormal, 50. *See also*
  Hallucinations, auditory

Perchloric acid extract, brain ^{31}P
  NMR spectrum of, **224,** 224
Performance Intelligence Quotient
  (PIQ), 96
Persecutory delusions, 52
Personality, premorbid, 6–7
PET. *See* Positron-emission
  tomography (PET)
Phase-specific strategies, for
  psychosocial treatment,
  205–207
Phencyclidine (PCP; angel dust),
  169–170
Phenomenology, 47–48. *See also*
  Symptoms
  problems in model development
    and, **51,** 51–53
Phenotype
  affected
    definition of, 252, 258
    classification by, 249–250
Phoniness, preoccupation with, 8
Phosphatidylcholine (PtdC), 222
Phosphatidylethanolamine (PtdE),
  222
Phosphatidylinositol (PtdI), 222
Phosphatidylserine (PtdS), 222
Phosphocholine, **224,** 224, 225, 226
Phosphocreatine (PCr)
  ^{31}P NMR study of, **224,** 224
  energy metabolism and, 228
  in vitro studies of, 226, 227
  in vivo studies of, 229, **231**
  ratio to inorganic orthophosphate,
    228, 229
Phosphodiester (PDE)
  ^{31}P NMR study of, **224,** 224
  in autistic patients, 235
  in early schizophrenia, neuro-
    trophic therapy for, 238
  in vivo studies of, 229
  resonances of, in mammalian
    brain, 228

Phosphodiesterase, decreased levels
in schizophrenia, causes of,
234–235
Phosphoethanolamine, 223, **224,**
224, 225, 226
Phospholipase A₁, 234–235
Phospholipase A₂, 222, 234–235
Phosphomonoester (PME). *See also*
α-GP; Phosphocholine;
Phosphoethanolamine
animal studies of, 226
in autistic patients, 235
decreased levels in schizophrenia,
causes of, 234–235
in early schizophrenia,
neurotrophic therapy for, 238
in vivo studies of, 229
ratio to PDE, 226–227
ratio to phosphodiester, 226–227
resonances of, in mammalian
brain, 228
Phosphorus-31 nuclear magnetic
resonance
in aging, 232–233
implications of studies, 236–238
in normal brain development,
232–233
in vitro studies, 223–228, **224**
in vitro vs. in vivo findings, 232
in vivo studies, **228–229, 230, 231,**
232
schizophrenic v. control subjects,
233–235
schizophrenic vs. autistic patients,
235
L-Phosphoserine, **224,** 224, 225
Pi. *See* Inorganic orthophosphate (Pi)
Piaget, J., genetic epistemology
theories of, 33
PIQ (Performance Intelligence
Quotient), 96
Platelet monoamine oxidase (MAO),
110

PME, *See* Phosphomonoester (PME)
PME-to-PDE ratio, in vivo studies of,
229
Pons, 135
Porteus Mazes, 79
Positive symptoms, 36
D₂ receptor density and, 126
D₂ receptor quantity and, 124–125
factor analysis studies of, **57,** 57
in leukotomized patients, 63–64,
65, 66
listing of, **56,** 57
SAPS, reliability coefficients for
items in, **60**
standardized evaluation techniques
for, 57–58
subdivisions, 57
Positron-emission tomography
(PET), 147
of autistic patients, 235
cameras, first, 148
clinical studies, first, 148
of D₁ receptor occupancy in
neuroleptic treatment,
182–183
of dopamine receptors, 150–153,
153–154
antipsychotic drug treatment
and, 151–153, **152**
of frontal metabolism, **75–78**
of regional brain energy
metabolism, 148–150
regional brain glucose metabolism,
during neuroleptic treatment,
150
of striatal D₂ receptor
concentration, 126
tracers for, 147–148
Postmortem studies
of brain stem, 135–136
of cerebral cortex, 133–135, **134**
of D₂ receptors in caudate and
putamen, 237

Postmortem studies (continued)
in vivo imaging and, 122, 123–124
of limbic system, 131–133
Postpsychotic depression,
psychosocial treatment strategies
for, 206
Poverty, schizophrenia and, 21, 23
3-PPP, 165, 165
Preferential dopaminergic
autoreceptor antagonists,
166–167
Prefrontal cortex
connections of, 59, 61, 61
decreased perfusion in, 69, 70–78,
79
dorsal, in vivo ^{31}P NMR imaging of,
230, 231
dorsolateral subdivision of, 61, 61
medial subdivision of, 61, 61
middle, 149
negative symptoms and, 59, 61,
61–62
orbital subdivision of, 61, 61
premature aging of, 238
Prefrontal glutamatergic pathway,
237–238
Prefrontal leukotomy, 62–63. See also
Leukotomized patients
Premorbid personality, 6–7
Preventive measures, 14–15
Primate animal models, 54
Prognosis, 7, 10, 35–36
Prognostic factors, 191
Programmed synaptic pruning,
236–237
Prolactin, clozapine and, 179
Propranolol, 182
N-n-Propyl-3-(3-hydroxyphenyl)
piperidine, 165, 165
Psychiatrist, perspective of, 12–16
Psychodynamic approach, vs.
biological psychiatry, 32–34
Psychological configurations, 37–38

Psychological factors, etiology and,
14–15
Psychometric studies, 48
methodological problems in, 96–98
Psychosis, depressive with mood-
incongruent delusions, 250
Psychosocial education, 13
Psychosocial factors
vicissitudes of schizophrenia and,
190–194
vulnerability-stress model and,
194–196
Psychosocial services
definition of, 198
goals of, 198–199
Psychosocial treatment, 189
historical landmarks in America
for, 209–213
outcome dimensions, 198–203
phase-specific strategies for, 205–207
principles, 204
strategies, general, 204–205
Psychoticism factor, 57
PtdC (phosphatidylcholine), 222
PtdE (phosphatidylethanolamine),
222
PtdI (phosphatidylinositol), 222
PtdS (phosphatidylserine), 222
Public mental health services, 22
Public misconceptions, 3
Public policy issues, 23–25
Public safety goals, 199
Public safety outcome dimensions,
202–203
Putamen
D2 receptors in, 124
number of D2 receptors, 125
serotonin in, 127

QNB, in cerebral cortex, 134

^{11}C-Raclopride, 150–152, 152
Radioisotopes

for PET tracers, 69, 147–148
for SPECT tracers, 69
Radiotracers. *See* Tracers
Rating scales, 51
Refusal of services, 203
Regional brain energy metabolism,
    in schizophrenia, 148–150
Rehabilitation, 199–200
    alternative living arrangements
        and, 17
    effect on family, 12
    goals of, 25, 199
    instrumental functioning outcome
        dimension of, 200–201
    social functioning outcome
        dimension of, 200
Relapse rates
    for family therapy, **208,** 208
    for family therapy and social skills
        training, **208,** 208
    high expressed emotion families
        and, 193
    for social skills training, **208,** 208
Research
    federal support for, 29–30
    investigations, replication
        problems of, 52
    outcome dimensions of, 198–203
Resources
    allocation of, 23
    existing, efficacy of, 29
Restriction fragment length
    polymorphisms (RFLPs), 220
Risperidone, 181

SADS (Schedule for Affective
    Disorders and Schizophrenia),
    233
SANS. *See* Scale for the Assessment of
    Negative Symptoms (SANS)
SAPS. *See* Scale for the Assessment of
    Positive Symptoms (SAPS)

Scale for the Assessment of Negative
    Symptoms (SANS), 80
    cultural settings and, **58,** 58
    global ratings for items in, **60**
    reliability coefficients for items in,
        60
Scale for the Assessment of Positive
    Symptoms (SAPS), 80
    cultural settings and, 58, 59
    global ratings for items in, **60**
    reliability coefficients for items in,
        60
Schedule for Affective Disorders and
    Schizophrenia (SADS), 233
Schedule of Schizotypal Personalities
    (SSP), 251
Schizoaffective disorder, 250, 251
Schizoid personality, with
    schizophrenia, 249
Schizophreniform disorder,
    250, 251
Schizotypal disorder, 251
Self-esteem, 41
Self-help, 25
Self-regulatory processes, 40
Senile dementia, neuroleptic-treated,
    D_2 receptor density in, 126
Sequential program, for studying
    mental illness, **55,** 55–56
Serotonin
    in cerebral cortex, **134**
    in lateral hypothalamus, 131
    in medulla, 135
    in mesencephalon, 135
    neuroleptics and, 180–181
    in putamen, 127
    uptake, 130
Setoperone, 180
Shame, 10
Siblings, supportive, 11
Sigma sites, 170
Signa system, 228
Signs, 47–48

Single photon emission computed
    tomography (SPECT)
  for cerebral blood flow
      measurement, 69
  of frontal metabolism in
      schizophrenia, **70–75**
  ligand in, 151
Social factors, etiology and, 14–15
Social functioning outcome
    dimensions, 200
Social networks, 191
Social relations functioning, 36
Social skills training, relapse rates for,
    208, 208
Socioeconomic factors, 190–191
Software programs, 17
Somatostatin, **134,** 136
SPECT. *See* Single photon emission
    computed tomography (SPECT)
Speech
  comprehension of, 54
  disorganized, 48, 50, 52, 57
  poverty of, 54
SRIF (somatostatin), **134,** 136
SSDI (supplemental security
    disability income), 22, 29
SSI (supplemental security income),
    22, 24, 29
SSP (Schedule of Schizotypal
    Personalities), 251
Stability of illness, 12
Standardized tests, 55–56
State government, 28–29
State mental health programs, 28
Stereotypy, apomorphine or ampheta-
    mine, clozapine, and, 179
Stigma of mental illness, 10
Stress
  dopamine release and, 238
  life event, 191–192
  psychopathology and, 33
  vulnerability-stress model and,
      194–196

Stria terminalis, bed nucleus of, 131
Striatum
  D2 receptor density, neuroleptics
      and, 179
  D2 receptors, 136
  D2 receptors in, 124–125
Stroop Color-Word Inference Test, for
    leukotomized patients, **67,** 67–69
Structured milieu therapy, 210–211
Subacute phase, psychosocial
    treatment strategies for, 206
Subcortical dementia, 95
Substantia nigra, GABAergic
    supersensitivity, 180
Suicidal ideation, 8
Sullivan, Harry Stack, 209–211,
    212–213
Supplemental security disability
    income (SSDI), 22, 29
Supplemental security income (SSI),
    22, 24, 29
Sydenham, T., 35
Symptoms. *See also* Phenomenology
  brain mechanisms of, 49–50
  brain structure/function and, 50–51
  clinical assessment of, 56–59
  definitions of, 51
  diversity of, 52
  identifying, 55
  loss of will, 37
  modeling, neurological vs.
      psychiatric presentation, 54
  multiple cognitive and behavioral
      domains, 52
  negative. *See* Negative symptoms
  positive. *See* Positive symptoms
  ratings for, 34–35
  reduction of, 160
  severity of, 36
  types of, 3, 11–12, 47–48
Synapse, 161
Synaptic pruning, programmed,
    236–237

Talking treatment, 211
Tardive dyskinesia, 163, 177, 179
  GABAergic functional involvement
    in, 180
Tardive dystonia, 177
Tefludazine, 180
Temporal lobe
  lesions of, 95
  magnetic resonance imaging of,
    111
Temporal lobe hypothesis
  selective impairment of, 98
  support for, 98
Test batteries, 100
Thalamus
  dorsomedial, 136
  gamma-aminobutyric acid in,
    135–136
Therapeutic window, 175
Third ventricle enlargement, 133
Thought
  abstract, 9
  delusional, 8, 9–10
  impoverished, 10
Thought disorder, positive formal
  disturbed function in, 56
  factor analysis studies of, 57
  modeling of, 54
Thyrotropin-releasing hormone
  (TRH), in cerebral cortex, 134
Time course of response, 176–177
Timing strategy, in psychosocial
  treatment, 205
Titration strategy, in psychosocial
  treatment, 205
Tower of London, 79, 80–81
Tracers
  for PET, 69, 147–148
  for SPECT, 69
Trail Making Test, for leukotomized
  patients, 67, 67–69
Treatment of schizophrenia,
  159–160

TRH (thyrotropin-releasing
    hormone), in cerebral cortex,
    134
Triplet study, 109
Twins
  environmental risk and, 109–115,
    110, 112, 113, 114, 115
  historical aspects, 105
  risks of, 114
  schizophrenia and, 115
  specific abnormalities of, 113
  studies of, 48, 116
    classic, 106, 107, 106–107
    hippocampus abnormalities and,
      132
    limitations for, 113
  susceptibility to schizophrenia,
    113–115

(+)-UH232, 166, 167, 167
  locomotor activity in rats and, 168,
    168
Unconditional love, 40
Uridine diphosphosugars, 225

Ventral septum, 131
Ventricular brain ratio (VBR),
  113
Ventricular enlargement. See
  Cerebral ventricular size
Verbal Intelligence Quotient (VIQ),
  96
Visual perception, 50
Vocational rehabilitation, 200
Vulnerability, to schizophrenia,
  194–195
Vulnerability-stress model, 194–196

Wechsler Memory Scale, 95
Wernicke's aphasia, vs.
  schizophrenia, 54
Will, loss of, 37

Wisconsin Card Sorting Test, 17
   executive function deficits and,
      94–95, 96
   frontal lobe hypothesis and, 98
   for leukotomized patients, **67,**
      67–68
   prefrontal cortex function and, 79

Withdrawal, emotional, 54
Woodshedding, 39–40

^{133}Xe method, for cerebral blood
   flow measurement, 80
X rays, 6